# Table of Contents

## Front Matter

## Chapter 1: Introduction to Moringa Oleifera

- Global Significance

# Chapter 2: What is Moringa Oleifera?

- Botanical Description
- Origin and Distribution
- Varieties and Species

# Chapter 3: Uses of Moringa

- Traditional Uses
- Modern Applications
- Global Adoption

# Chapter 4: Benefits of Moringa

- Nutritional Benefits
- Health Benefits
- Environmental Benefits

# Chapter 5: How Moringa Has Helped People

- Personal Testimonials
- Case Studies
- Community Impact Stories

# Chapter 6: Nutritional Value of Moringa

- Comprehensive Nutrient Profile
- Comparison with Other Superfoods
- Bioavailability of Nutrients

# Chapter 7: How It's Grown, Where It's Grown

- Cultivation Requirements
- Global Growing Regions
- Cultivation Techniques

# Chapter 8: Moringa for Detox

- Detoxification Properties
- Liver Health Benefits
- Detox Protocols and Methods

# Chapter 9: How Moringa Heals and Energizes

- Medicinal Properties
- Energy-Boosting Effects
- Healing Applications

# Chapter 10: Frequently Asked Questions

- Common Questions and Concerns
- Expert Answers
- Usage Guidelines

# Chapter 11: Latest Scientific Research on Moringa

- Recent Discoveries
- Clinical Studies
- Emerging Applications

# Chapter 12: Advanced Cultivation Techniques for Moringa

- Climate-Specific Growing Methods
- Soil Preparation and Management
- Pest and Disease Control
- Harvesting and Processing

# Chapter 13: Global Perspectives on Moringa Use

- Regional Variations in Cultivation and Consumption
- Cultural Significance in Different Countries
- International Development Projects

# Chapter 14: Moringa in Modern Healthcare

- Integration with Conventional Medicine
- Practitioner Perspectives
- Patient Experiences and Case Studies
- Dosage Guidelines and Safety Considerations

# Chapter 15: Sustainable Farming and Economic Impact of Moringa

- Moringa as a Sustainable Crop
- Economic Opportunities Along the Value Chain
- Fair Trade and Ethical Sourcing
- Case Studies of Successful Moringa Enterprises

# Back Matter

- References
- Resources for Further Information
- Index

# CHAPTER 1

## INTRODUCTION TO MORINGA OLEIFERA

Welcome to the remarkable world of Moringa oleifera, a plant that has earned its reputation as the "miracle tree" through centuries of traditional use and, more recently, through rigorous scientific validation. This extraordinary plant offers a rare combination of nutritional excellence, medicinal properties, and environmental benefits that make it uniquely valuable in our modern world.

# What is Moringa?

Moringa oleifera is a fast-growing, drought-resistant tree native to the foothills of the Himalayas in northwestern India but now cultivated throughout the tropics and subtropics worldwide. Distinguished by its delicate, feathery leaves and uniquely shaped seed pods, this resilient tree has adapted to thrive in challenging environments where many other plants struggle to survive.

What truly sets Moringa apart, however, is not just its hardiness but its exceptional nutritional profile. Often described as "nature's multivitamin," Moringa leaves contain remarkable concentrations of vitamins, minerals, amino acids, and beneficial plant compounds. Gram for gram, these unassuming green leaves provide more vitamin A than carrots, more calcium than milk, more iron than spinach, more vitamin C than oranges, and more potassium than bananas.

Beyond nutrition, every part of the Moringa tree—from roots to seeds—offers valuable applications. The seeds purify water, the oil moisturizes skin, the roots treat inflammatory conditions, and the leaves address dozens of health concerns from diabetes to malnutrition. This versatility has earned Moringa many names across cultures: "drumstick tree" for its long seed pods, "horseradish tree" for its root flavor, and most tellingly, "tree of life" for its life-sustaining properties.

## Historical Background

The story of Moringa stretches back thousands of years, woven into the fabric of ancient civilizations. Archaeological evidence suggests that Moringa was valued in the Indus Valley

Civilization over 4,000 years ago, where it likely served both nutritional and medicinal purposes.

In ancient Egypt, Moringa oil—extracted from the seeds—was so prized that it was placed in tombs with pharaohs for use in the afterlife. The Egyptians valued this "Ben oil" (as it was known) for its resistance to rancidity, its use in perfumes, and its ability to protect skin from the harsh desert environment.

Ancient Greek and Roman physicians documented Moringa's medicinal properties, with references appearing in medical texts from the first century AD. These early Western healers recognized the plant's anti-inflammatory properties and prescribed it for a variety of ailments.

In traditional Ayurvedic medicine of India, Moringa has been documented for over 4,000 years. Ayurvedic texts cite Moringa as a remedy for over 300 diseases, describing specific applications for different parts of the plant. This sophisticated understanding of Moringa's varied properties demonstrates the depth of traditional knowledge developed through centuries of observation and clinical experience.

Indigenous healing traditions across Africa and the Americas similarly incorporated Moringa after its introduction to these regions, developing their own applications based on local health needs and cultural contexts. This cross-cultural adoption speaks to the plant's universal value and adaptability.

## Global Significance

Today, Moringa's significance extends far beyond its historical uses, addressing some of our most pressing global challenges. In regions facing malnutrition, Moringa provides accessible, locally-grown nutrition that can literally save lives. International organizations including the World Health Organization and the Food and Agriculture Organization have promoted Moringa cultivation as a natural solution to malnutrition, particularly for pregnant women, nursing mothers, and young children.

In our environmental crisis, Moringa offers multiple ecological benefits. Its drought resistance makes it valuable in regions experiencing climate change-induced water scarcity. Its rapid growth allows for carbon sequestration, while its deep roots prevent soil erosion. When planted in agroforestry systems, Moringa enhances biodiversity and soil health while providing sustainable livelihoods.

Economically, Moringa creates opportunities along its entire value chain—from cultivation and processing to distribution and retail. In rural communities across Africa and Asia, Moringa enterprises provide income for farmers, processors, and entrepreneurs, with particular benefits for women who often lead these initiatives.

In the wellness sector, Moringa has emerged as a leading superfood, with global demand growing at over 8% annually. This market growth creates economic opportunities while introducing more people to Moringa's benefits. Scientific research continues to validate traditional uses while discovering new applications, from water purification to sustainable biofuel production.

Perhaps most importantly, Moringa represents a bridge between traditional wisdom and modern science—demonstrating how ancient knowledge, when subjected to scientific inquiry, often reveals solutions to contemporary problems. In a world increasingly recognizing the limitations of technological quick-fixes, Moringa reminds us that some of our most valuable resources have been hiding in plain sight for millennia.

As you explore this book, you'll discover the many dimensions of this extraordinary plant—from its nutritional composition to its medicinal applications, from cultivation techniques to economic opportunities. Whether you're approaching Moringa as a health enthusiast, a gardener, a healthcare practitioner, or simply a curious reader, this remarkable tree has something valuable to offer. Welcome to the world of Moringa oleifera—nature's gift to humanity.

# CHAPTER 2

## WHAT IS MORINGA OLEIFERA?

Moringa oleifera stands as one of nature's most remarkable botanical treasures—a plant whose extraordinary properties have earned it descriptive names like "miracle tree" and "tree of life" across cultures and continents. This chapter explores the botanical characteristics, origin, distribution, and varieties of this exceptional plant, providing a foundation for understanding its diverse applications and benefits.

## Botanical Description

Moringa oleifera is a fast-growing, deciduous tree belonging to the family Moringaceae. When allowed to grow naturally, it can reach heights of 10-12 meters (32-40 feet), though it is often pruned to maintain a more manageable height for harvesting. The trunk is typically straight but can sometimes be poorly formed, with a diameter reaching up to 45 centimeters (18 inches) at maturity.

The tree's most distinctive feature is its compound leaves, which are arranged feather-like (pinnate) with small leaflets. These delicate, oval-shaped leaflets are approximately 1-2 centimeters long, giving the foliage an elegant, fern-like appearance. The leaves are a vibrant green, providing a visual indication of their rich nutritional content.

Moringa produces fragrant, cream-colored flowers arranged in drooping panicles. These five-petaled blossoms measure about 2.5 centimeters in diameter and appear in clusters, creating a visually striking display when the tree is in bloom. In favorable conditions, Moringa can flower throughout the year, though flowering is often more prolific during certain seasons depending on the local climate.

Perhaps the most recognizable part of the Moringa tree is its distinctive seed pods, often called "drumsticks" due to their long, slender, stick-like appearance. These three-sided pods typically grow 30-45 centimeters (12-18 inches) in length, though some varieties produce pods up to 120 centimeters (4 feet) long. Young pods are green, tender, and edible, while mature pods turn brown and woody, containing the round seeds within.

The seeds themselves are remarkable—about 1 centimeter in diameter with three papery wings that aid in dispersal. Each tree can produce between 15,000 and 25,000 seeds annually. The roots of the Moringa tree are equally distinctive, with the main taproot resembling a horseradish root in appearance and flavor, which explains another common name: "horseradish tree."

## Origin and Distribution

Moringa oleifera is native to the sub-Himalayan regions of northern India, particularly in the states of Uttar Pradesh, Bihar, and Punjab. Archaeological evidence suggests that it has been cultivated in this region for at least 4,000 years, with ancient texts documenting its medicinal uses dating back to early Ayurvedic traditions.

From its Indian homeland, Moringa spread throughout Asia, likely through trade routes and cultural exchanges. It reached Southeast Asia centuries ago, becoming integrated into local food systems and traditional medicine practices in countries like the Philippines, Indonesia, and Thailand.

The plant's journey to Africa likely began around the 1st century AD through trade across the Indian Ocean. In East Africa, particularly in countries like Kenya and Tanzania, Moringa became established early on. Its spread to West Africa occurred later but was equally significant, with the plant becoming an important nutritional resource in countries like Ghana, Nigeria, and Senegal.

European colonization facilitated Moringa's introduction to the Caribbean and Latin America in the 18th and 19th centuries. In countries like Haiti, Jamaica, and Mexico, it found favorable growing conditions and was gradually incorporated into local cuisines and healing traditions.

Today, Moringa oleifera grows throughout the tropical and subtropical regions of the world, from Asia and Africa to Latin America and the Caribbean. Its remarkable adaptability to different soil types and climatic conditions has enabled its widespread distribution. While it thrives best in hot, semi-arid tropical climates, it has demonstrated impressive resilience in various environments, contributing to its global presence.

In recent decades, awareness of Moringa's nutritional and medicinal properties has sparked renewed interest in its cultivation, even in regions outside its traditional growing areas. With climate change creating new challenges for agriculture, Moringa's drought resistance and nutritional density have made it increasingly valuable for food security initiatives worldwide.

## Varieties and Species

While Moringa oleifera is the most widely known and cultivated species of the genus, the Moringa family (Moringaceae) includes 13 distinct species, each with unique characteristics and native ranges:

1. **Moringa oleifera**: The most common and widely distributed species, native to India but now cultivated globally.
2. **Moringa stenopetala**: Often called the African Moringa, this species is native to Ethiopia and Kenya. It produces larger leaves than M. oleifera and is particularly drought-resistant, making it valuable in arid regions.

3.  **Moringa peregrina**: Native to the Red Sea area, Arabian Peninsula, and Horn of Africa, this species is known for its exceptional oil quality and medicinal properties.

4.  **Moringa drouhardii**: Endemic to Madagascar, this species is distinguished by its bottle-shaped trunk that stores water, an adaptation to the island's seasonal dry periods.

5.  **Moringa hildebrandtii**: Another Madagascar native, this species can grow up to 25 meters tall, making it the largest in the Moringa family.

6.  **Moringa arborea**: Found in northeastern Kenya, this rare species was only scientifically described in 2001, highlighting that our knowledge of the Moringa family continues to evolve.

7.  **Moringa rivae**: Native to Kenya and Ethiopia, this species thrives in rocky, mountainous terrain.

8.  **Moringa borziana**: Found in Somalia and Kenya, this species has adapted to extremely arid conditions.

9.  **Moringa pygmaea**: As its name suggests, this is the smallest Moringa species, growing as a small shrub in Somalia.

10. **Moringa longituba**: Native to Kenya, Ethiopia, and Somalia, this species produces tuberous roots that help it survive drought.

11. **Moringa ovalifolia**: Found in Namibia and Angola, this species has a distinctive swollen trunk similar to a baobab tree.

12. **Moringa concanensis**: Native to India and Pakistan, this species is sometimes used as a rootstock for M. oleifera in commercial cultivation.

13.    **Moringa ruspoliana**: Native to Ethiopia, Kenya, and Somalia, this species is adapted to arid conditions and produces edible leaves.

Within Moringa oleifera itself, several cultivars have been developed through selective breeding to enhance specific characteristics:

- **PKM-1**: Developed in India, this cultivar is known for high pod production and is widely grown for vegetable purposes.
- **PKM-2**: An improved version of PKM-1 with higher yield potential and disease resistance.
- **Jaffna**: A cultivar from Sri Lanka known for its short pods and distinctive flavor.
- **Chavakacheri Murunga**: Another Sri Lankan variety prized for its taste and texture.
- **Chemmurunga**: A Kerala, India variety with particularly tender pods.
- **Yadhrasthic**: Developed for leaf production rather than pod production, this cultivar produces abundant, nutritious foliage.

Research institutions and agricultural organizations continue to develop new Moringa varieties adapted to specific growing conditions and end uses. Some breeding programs focus on enhancing nutritional content, while others prioritize drought resistance, pest tolerance, or growth rate. This ongoing development ensures that Moringa cultivation can be optimized for diverse environments and purposes.

## Conclusion

Moringa oleifera represents a botanical marvel whose unique characteristics have made it valuable across cultures and continents. Its distinctive morphology—from feathery leaves to drumstick-shaped pods—makes it easily recognizable, while its remarkable adaptability has enabled its global spread from its Indian homeland.

The diversity within the Moringa family, encompassing 13 species adapted to various ecological niches, demonstrates nature's ingenuity in evolving plants suited to challenging environments. As climate change creates new agricultural challenges, this adaptability becomes increasingly valuable.

Understanding Moringa's botanical characteristics, origin, distribution, and varieties provides essential context for appreciating its numerous applications and benefits. Whether viewed through the lens of traditional knowledge systems that have valued it for millennia or modern scientific research that continues to uncover its properties, Moringa oleifera stands as a testament to the extraordinary resources that the plant kingdom offers humanity.

# CHAPTER 3

## USES OF MORINGA

Moringa oleifera stands as one of the most versatile plants on our planet, with applications spanning nutrition, medicine, agriculture, water purification, and more. This chapter explores the remarkable range of uses for this extraordinary tree, from ancient traditional practices to innovative modern applications.

# Traditional Uses

Throughout history, communities across Asia, Africa, and beyond have developed sophisticated knowledge of Moringa's diverse applications, passing this wisdom through generations.

## Culinary Traditions

In South Asian cuisine, particularly in India, Moringa has been a dietary staple for thousands of years. The young seed pods, known as "drumsticks," are prized ingredients in curries, sambars, and other traditional dishes. These tender pods are typically cut into sections and cooked until soft, with diners extracting the nutritious pulp and seeds by pulling the pieces between their teeth —a distinctive eating experience that has become part of the cultural fabric.

The leaves feature prominently in many regional cuisines as well. In the Philippines, Moringa leaves (known locally as "malunggay") are essential ingredients in tinola, a traditional chicken soup believed to boost the milk production of nursing mothers. In Haiti, Moringa leaves are added to soup joumou, a celebratory dish with deep historical significance tied to the country's independence.

In West African traditions, dried Moringa leaf powder is incorporated into sauces and stews, providing essential nutrients during seasonal food scarcity. This practice represents indigenous nutritional wisdom that long predated scientific understanding of vitamins and minerals.

**Traditional Medicine Systems**

Ayurveda, India's ancient medical system dating back over 5,000 years, recognizes Moringa as a powerful medicinal plant with applications for treating over 300 conditions. Ayurvedic practitioners use different parts of the tree for specific purposes: roots for inflammation, bark for digestive issues, leaves for balancing blood sugar, and seeds for purifying water and treating skin conditions.

In Traditional Chinese Medicine, Moringa (known as "la mu") was introduced later but became valued for its warming properties and ability to clear stagnation in the body. Practitioners particularly noted its benefits for joint pain, digestive disorders, and edema.

Across Africa, traditional healers have incorporated Moringa into their pharmacopeia, developing unique applications based on local health needs. In Nigeria, for example, traditional birth attendants have long recommended Moringa to pregnant and nursing women to support maternal and infant health—a practice now validated by nutritional science.

**Household and Community Applications**

Beyond food and medicine, traditional communities found numerous practical applications for Moringa:

The oil extracted from Moringa seeds, known as Ben oil, has been used for centuries in perfumery and as a skin moisturizer. Its resistance to rancidity made it particularly valuable in hot climates before modern preservation methods.

The seed cake remaining after oil extraction has traditionally been used as a natural fertilizer, returning nutrients to the soil and improving crop yields—an early form of sustainable agriculture.

Perhaps most remarkably, crushed Moringa seeds have been used for water purification in Africa for centuries. Rural communities discovered that adding crushed seeds to turbid water causes impurities to bind together and settle, resulting in clearer, safer drinking water—a traditional practice that modern science has confirmed and refined.

## Modern Applications

Building on traditional knowledge, contemporary science and innovation have expanded Moringa's applications across numerous fields.

### Nutritional Supplements

In today's global marketplace, Moringa has emerged as a leading superfood, available in various forms:

Moringa leaf powder, the most common supplement form, provides a concentrated source of nutrients that can be added to smoothies, juices, or foods. With its complete amino acid profile and rich micronutrient content, it offers a plant-based nutritional boost particularly valued by vegetarians and vegans.

Capsules provide a convenient, tasteless option for those who find the distinctive flavor of Moringa challenging. These standardized doses make it easier to incorporate Moringa into daily wellness routines.

Moringa tea, made from dried leaves, offers a milder way to enjoy the plant's benefits while providing antioxidants and anti-inflammatory compounds. Some commercial blends combine Moringa with complementary herbs to enhance flavor and target specific health concerns.

Energy bars, protein powders, and other functional foods increasingly feature Moringa as manufacturers respond to consumer demand for nutrient-dense, plant-based ingredients with proven health benefits.

**Pharmaceutical and Cosmetic Applications**

The pharmaceutical industry has taken note of Moringa's medicinal properties, leading to various applications:

Standardized extracts targeting specific health conditions are being developed and tested in clinical trials. These include formulations for managing diabetes, hypertension, and inflammatory conditions, with promising early results.

Wound-healing products incorporating Moringa extract capitalize on its antimicrobial and anti-inflammatory properties. These range from hospital-grade dressings to consumer products for minor cuts and abrasions.

The cosmetics industry has embraced Moringa oil as a premium ingredient in skincare products. Its high oleic acid content makes it deeply moisturizing, while its antioxidants help protect skin from environmental damage. Major beauty brands now feature Moringa in everything from facial serums to hair conditioners.

Moringa-based oral care products, including toothpaste and mouthwash, utilize the plant's antimicrobial properties to fight plaque and gingivitis while providing a natural alternative to synthetic ingredients.

## Agricultural Applications

Modern agricultural systems are finding valuable applications for Moringa beyond direct human consumption:

As animal feed, Moringa leaves provide exceptional nutrition for livestock and poultry. Studies show that adding even small amounts of Moringa to animal diets can improve growth rates, milk production, and overall health while reducing the need for synthetic supplements.

Biopesticides derived from Moringa offer farmers natural alternatives to chemical pest control. Compounds in the leaves and seeds have demonstrated effectiveness against various crop pests while posing minimal environmental risks.

Biofertilizers made from Moringa enhance soil fertility and plant growth. The seed cake left after oil extraction is particularly valuable, providing nutrients and improving soil structure when applied to agricultural fields.

Green manure applications involve planting Moringa as a cover crop, then incorporating the biomass into the soil to improve fertility. This practice enhances soil organic matter, microbial activity, and water retention capacity.

## Environmental Applications

Moringa's environmental applications address some of today's most pressing ecological challenges:

Water purification systems using Moringa seed extract have been developed for both community-scale and industrial applications. These systems capitalize on the natural coagulant properties of Moringa proteins to remove turbidity and reduce bacterial contamination in water supplies.

Phytoremediation projects utilize Moringa's ability to absorb heavy metals and other contaminants from soil. By planting Moringa in polluted areas, environmental engineers can gradually reduce soil toxicity while producing valuable biomass.

Agroforestry systems incorporate Moringa as a multifunctional tree that provides shade for other crops, prevents soil erosion, fixes nitrogen, and produces nutritious leaves and pods. These integrated systems enhance biodiversity while maximizing land productivity.

Biofuel production represents another promising application, with Moringa oil showing potential as a biodiesel feedstock. Unlike some biofuel crops, Moringa can be grown on marginal land not suitable for food production, avoiding the food-versus-fuel dilemma.

## Global Adoption

The uses of Moringa have spread globally, with different regions adapting applications to local needs and contexts.

### Humanitarian Applications

International development organizations have embraced Moringa as a tool for addressing malnutrition and food insecurity:

School feeding programs in countries including Ghana, Nicaragua, and Haiti incorporate Moringa powder into meals, significantly improving the nutritional value of children's diets. These programs often include educational components teaching children and parents about Moringa cultivation and use.

Maternal health initiatives provide Moringa supplements to pregnant and lactating women in regions with high rates of maternal malnutrition. These programs aim to improve birth outcomes and infant health while empowering women with knowledge about nutrition.

Emergency response organizations increasingly include Moringa in their nutritional interventions during humanitarian crises. Its long shelf life, concentrated nutrition, and cultural acceptability in many regions make it particularly valuable in emergency contexts.

## Commercial and Economic Applications

The growing global market for Moringa has created economic opportunities along the entire value chain:

Smallholder farming initiatives focused on Moringa cultivation provide sustainable livelihoods for rural communities. Organizations like Kuli Kuli in the United States partner with farmer cooperatives in developing countries to ensure fair compensation and sustainable practices.

Value-added processing creates jobs and economic opportunities beyond primary production. From simple solar drying operations to sophisticated extraction facilities, Moringa processing adds value locally rather than exporting raw materials.

Export markets for Moringa products continue to expand as awareness of its benefits grows in North America, Europe, and East Asia. This global demand creates economic incentives for sustainable cultivation and quality control.

## Conclusion

The remarkable diversity of Moringa's uses—spanning nutrition, medicine, agriculture, and environmental applications—makes it uniquely valuable in addressing multiple contemporary challenges. From traditional wisdom that recognized its healing properties centuries ago to cutting-edge research uncovering new applications, Moringa continues to demonstrate its extraordinary versatility.

What makes Moringa particularly significant is how it bridges traditional knowledge and modern science, rural livelihoods and global markets, simple household uses and sophisticated industrial applications. Few plants offer such a wide range of benefits while growing in challenging conditions where many other species fail.

As we face complex challenges including climate change, food insecurity, water scarcity, and public health crises, Moringa's diverse applications offer sustainable solutions that honor traditional wisdom while embracing scientific innovation. The continued exploration of this remarkable plant's potential promises to reveal even more ways in which the "miracle tree" can benefit humanity and our planet.

# CHAPTER 4

## BENEFITS OF MORINGA

Moringa oleifera offers an extraordinary range of benefits that span nutritional, medicinal, environmental, and economic domains. This chapter explores these diverse advantages, examining how this remarkable plant contributes to human health, ecological sustainability, and community development worldwide.

### Nutritional Benefits

Moringa's nutritional profile is nothing short of exceptional, earning it recognition as one of nature's most complete superfoods.

## Comprehensive Nutrient Density

The leaves of Moringa oleifera contain an impressive concentration of essential nutrients that surpass many common foods:

Vitamin A, crucial for vision, immune function, and cellular communication, is present in Moringa leaves at levels four times higher than in carrots. This makes Moringa particularly valuable in regions where vitamin A deficiency causes preventable blindness and compromised immunity.

Calcium, essential for bone health, nerve transmission, and muscle function, appears in Moringa leaves at concentrations four times greater than in milk. This plant-based calcium source is especially beneficial for those who avoid dairy products or lack access to them.

Iron, necessary for oxygen transport in the blood and energy production, exists in Moringa leaves at levels three times higher than in spinach. This makes Moringa an excellent resource for preventing and addressing iron-deficiency anemia, particularly among women and children in developing regions.

Vitamin C, important for immune function, collagen synthesis, and iron absorption, is found in Moringa leaves at concentrations seven times greater than in oranges. This high vitamin C content not only supports immune health but also enhances the absorption of the plant's abundant iron.

Potassium, critical for heart function, fluid balance, and muscle contractions, appears in Moringa leaves at levels three times higher than in bananas. This essential mineral helps maintain healthy blood pressure and cardiovascular function.

## Complete Protein Source

Unlike most plant foods, Moringa leaves contain all nine essential amino acids, making them a complete protein source comparable to animal products:

The protein content in dried Moringa leaf powder ranges from 24-27%, rivaling that of eggs and exceeding many legumes. This high-quality protein is particularly valuable for vegetarians, vegans, and communities with limited access to animal protein sources.

The amino acid profile of Moringa protein is well-balanced, providing the building blocks necessary for tissue repair, enzyme production, and overall growth and development. This makes Moringa especially valuable for children, pregnant women, and those recovering from illness or injury.

The digestibility of Moringa protein exceeds that of many plant proteins, ensuring that the body can effectively utilize the amino acids it provides. Studies show that Moringa protein has a digestibility score of approximately 90%, comparable to many animal proteins.

## Essential Fatty Acids

Moringa seeds yield an oil rich in beneficial fatty acids that support multiple aspects of health:

Oleic acid, a monounsaturated fatty acid also found in olive oil, comprises approximately 70% of Moringa seed oil. This heart-healthy fat helps maintain healthy cholesterol levels and supports cardiovascular function.

The oil contains an ideal ratio of omega-6 to omega-3 fatty acids, promoting balanced inflammatory responses in the body. This balanced ratio contrasts with the excessive omega-6 content common in modern diets, which can contribute to chronic inflammation.

The stability of Moringa oil is remarkable, with high resistance to oxidation and rancidity due to its natural antioxidant content. This stability makes it valuable both for culinary applications and for cosmetic and medicinal uses.

**Micronutrient Powerhouse**

Beyond the major nutrients, Moringa provides an impressive array of micronutrients essential for optimal health:

The leaves contain over 46 antioxidants that protect cells from oxidative damage and reduce inflammation. These include quercetin, kaempferol, and various polyphenols that have been linked to reduced risk of chronic diseases.

Moringa provides rare plant-based sources of vitamins B1, B2, B3, and E, supporting energy metabolism, nervous system function, and cellular protection. This comprehensive vitamin profile makes Moringa particularly valuable in addressing multiple nutrient deficiencies simultaneously.

Trace minerals including zinc, magnesium, selenium, and copper are present in bioavailable forms, supporting immune function, enzyme activity, and antioxidant systems. These minerals play crucial roles in hundreds of biochemical processes throughout the body.

# Health Benefits

Scientific research continues to validate traditional knowledge about Moringa's medicinal properties, revealing mechanisms behind its diverse health benefits.

## Anti-inflammatory and Antioxidant Effects

Moringa contains powerful compounds that combat inflammation and oxidative stress:

Isothiocyanates, particularly moringin, demonstrate potent anti-inflammatory activity comparable to some pharmaceutical anti-inflammatories but without the side effects. These compounds inhibit inflammatory pathways and reduce the production of pro-inflammatory cytokines.

The antioxidant capacity of Moringa leaves, measured by ORAC (Oxygen Radical Absorbance Capacity), exceeds that of most common fruits and vegetables. This antioxidant power helps neutralize free radicals that contribute to aging and disease development.

Flavonoids including quercetin, kaempferol, and myricetin provide targeted anti-inflammatory benefits for specific tissues and systems. Research indicates these compounds may be particularly beneficial for respiratory and digestive inflammation.

## Blood Sugar Regulation

Moringa offers multiple mechanisms that support healthy glucose metabolism:

Chlorogenic acid and other polyphenols in Moringa leaves help regulate glucose absorption in the intestines, preventing rapid spikes in blood sugar after meals. This gradual absorption pattern is particularly beneficial for those with insulin resistance or diabetes.

Isothiocyanates influence insulin signaling pathways, potentially improving cellular sensitivity to insulin. This enhanced sensitivity allows cells to more effectively take up glucose from the bloodstream, reducing circulating blood sugar levels.

Fiber content in Moringa leaves slows carbohydrate digestion and absorption, contributing to more stable blood glucose levels. This effect helps prevent the energy crashes and cravings associated with rapid blood sugar fluctuations.

**Cardiovascular Support**

Research indicates that Moringa supports heart health through multiple mechanisms:

Regular consumption may help maintain healthy cholesterol levels by reducing LDL (low-density lipoprotein) cholesterol while supporting HDL (high-density lipoprotein) cholesterol. This favorable lipid profile reduces risk factors for atherosclerosis and heart disease.

The potassium content helps regulate blood pressure by balancing sodium levels and supporting proper fluid balance. This electrolyte balance is crucial for maintaining healthy blood pressure and reducing strain on the cardiovascular system.

Antioxidants in Moringa protect blood vessels from oxidative damage, maintaining their flexibility and function. This vascular protection is essential for overall cardiovascular health and circulation.

## Liver Support and Detoxification

Moringa provides valuable support for the body's primary detoxification organ:

Phytochemicals in Moringa leaves enhance Phase I and Phase II liver detoxification pathways, helping the body process and eliminate environmental toxins, medications, and metabolic waste products. This enhanced detoxification capacity supports overall health and vitality.

Studies show that Moringa extract can help protect liver cells from damage caused by toxins and medications. This hepatoprotective effect may be particularly valuable for those exposed to environmental pollutants or taking necessary but potentially hepatotoxic medications.

The anti-inflammatory compounds in Moringa help reduce liver inflammation, supporting recovery from conditions like fatty liver disease and hepatitis. This anti-inflammatory action complements the plant's detoxification support.

## Immune System Enhancement

Moringa provides comprehensive support for immune function:

The rich vitamin A content supports the integrity of mucous membranes that form the body's first line of defense against pathogens. These healthy barriers in the respiratory, digestive, and urogenital tracts prevent pathogen entry and colonization.

Vitamin C, zinc, and selenium work synergistically to support both innate and adaptive immune responses. This nutrient combination enhances the function of immune cells while supporting the production of antibodies.

Antimicrobial compounds in Moringa, including pterygospermin and benzyl isothiocyanate, demonstrate activity against various bacteria and fungi. These natural antimicrobials may help the body combat infections while supporting the balance of beneficial microorganisms.

## Environmental Benefits

Beyond human health, Moringa offers remarkable environmental advantages that address pressing ecological challenges.

### Soil Improvement and Erosion Control

Moringa contributes significantly to soil health and conservation:

The deep root system penetrates compacted soil layers, improving aeration and water infiltration. This soil conditioning effect benefits not only the Moringa tree but also surrounding plants and soil organisms.

Nitrogen-fixing bacteria associated with Moringa roots convert atmospheric nitrogen into forms available to plants, enhancing soil fertility naturally. This biological nitrogen fixation reduces the need for synthetic fertilizers while improving soil health.

When planted on slopes and degraded lands, Moringa's extensive root network helps prevent soil erosion by binding soil particles and reducing water runoff. This erosion control function is particularly valuable in regions experiencing deforestation and land degradation.

## Water Purification

Moringa seeds contain remarkable water-purifying properties:

The cationic proteins in Moringa seeds act as natural coagulants, binding to impurities in water and causing them to clump together for easy removal. This natural purification method can reduce water turbidity by 90-99% in properly treated water.

Antimicrobial properties in the seeds reduce bacterial contamination in water by 90-99.9% when used correctly. This reduction in pathogenic microorganisms significantly decreases the risk of waterborne diseases.

Unlike chemical water treatments, Moringa seed powder is biodegradable and produces minimal environmental impact. This makes it an ecologically sound option for water treatment, particularly in regions lacking infrastructure for conventional water purification.

## Climate Resilience and Carbon Sequestration

Moringa contributes to climate change mitigation and adaptation:

The rapid growth rate allows Moringa to sequester carbon dioxide quickly, with mature trees capturing an estimated 12-25 tons of carbon per hectare annually. This carbon sequestration helps mitigate greenhouse gas emissions contributing to climate change.

Drought resistance makes Moringa valuable in regions experiencing increasing water scarcity due to climate change. The tree can survive extended dry periods while continuing to provide nutritional and economic benefits to communities.

Agroforestry systems incorporating Moringa create microclimates that protect more sensitive crops from extreme temperatures and weather events. This protective function enhances agricultural resilience in the face of climate variability.

**Biodiversity Support**

Moringa plantings can enhance local biodiversity:

Flowering Moringa trees attract pollinators including bees, butterflies, and birds, supporting these essential species and the ecosystem services they provide. The extended flowering period of Moringa provides nectar resources when other plants may not be blooming.

Multi-layered agroforestry systems with Moringa create diverse habitats that support a range of beneficial insects, birds, and soil organisms. This biodiversity contributes to natural pest control and enhanced ecosystem function.

As a non-invasive species in most regions where it's cultivated, Moringa provides ecological benefits without the risks associated with invasive exotic plants. This makes it a responsible choice for agroforestry and reforestation projects.

# Economic Benefits

Moringa cultivation creates economic opportunities that support sustainable development and poverty reduction.

## Sustainable Livelihoods

Moringa enterprises provide income generation opportunities across the value chain:

Small-scale farmers benefit from Moringa's multiple harvests per year, providing more consistent income than seasonal crops. A single hectare of intensively managed Moringa can generate $15,000-$30,000 in annual revenue, depending on market access and processing capacity.

Processing operations create employment in rural areas where job opportunities are often limited. These jobs range from basic processing roles to skilled positions in quality control, management, and marketing.

Women often lead Moringa enterprises, from cultivation to product development, enhancing their economic independence and decision-making power. The flexibility of many Moringa-related activities allows women to balance income generation with household responsibilities.

## Low Investment Requirements

Moringa enterprises can start with minimal capital:

Seeds or cuttings are inexpensive and readily available in most tropical and subtropical regions. A small nursery can be established with basic materials and scaled up as resources permit.

Cultivation requires minimal inputs once established, with trees producing leaves without irrigation in many regions and requiring little or no fertilizer when grown in suitable soil. This low-input requirement reduces financial risk for resource-constrained farmers.

Simple processing methods like solar drying can be implemented with minimal equipment, allowing producers to add value to their harvest without significant capital investment. As businesses grow, more sophisticated processing can be gradually introduced.

## Multiple Revenue Streams

Moringa offers diverse income opportunities from a single crop:

Leaf production provides regular income through multiple harvests per year, with leaves sold fresh, dried, or processed into powder. This frequent harvesting cycle creates steady cash flow throughout the year.

Seed production represents another revenue stream, with mature trees producing 15,000-25,000 seeds annually. These seeds can be sold for propagation, oil extraction, or water purification applications.

Value-added products including oils, teas, capsules, and cosmetics allow producers to capture more value from their harvest. These products typically command higher prices than raw materials, increasing profit margins for producers.

## Conclusion

The benefits of Moringa oleifera extend far beyond any single dimension, encompassing nutritional excellence, medicinal properties, environmental contributions, and economic opportunities. This remarkable convergence of benefits in a single plant explains why Moringa has been revered across cultures and why it continues to attract increasing attention in our contemporary world.

What makes Moringa particularly valuable is how its benefits address multiple interconnected challenges simultaneously. Its nutritional density helps combat malnutrition while its environmental resilience supports climate adaptation. Its economic opportunities empower communities while its medicinal properties support public health. Few plants offer such comprehensive solutions to pressing human and ecological needs.

As we face complex global challenges including climate change, food insecurity, water scarcity, and public health crises, Moringa's diverse benefits offer sustainable solutions that honor traditional wisdom while embracing scientific innovation. The continued exploration of this remarkable plant's potential promises to reveal even more ways in which the "miracle tree" can benefit humanity and our planet.

# CHAPTER 5

## HOW MORINGA HAS HELPED PEOPLE

The true measure of Moringa's value lies not just in laboratory findings or nutritional analyses, but in the tangible ways it has transformed lives around the world. This chapter explores real-world examples of how Moringa oleifera has helped individuals and communities address health challenges, improve nutrition, and create sustainable livelihoods.

# Personal Health Transformations

Across continents and cultures, individuals have experienced remarkable health improvements through Moringa consumption, often when conventional approaches fell short.

## Recovery Stories

Maria's journey with chronic fatigue illustrates Moringa's potential for restoring vitality. After struggling with debilitating fatigue for three years following a viral infection, this 42-year-old teacher from Mexico began incorporating Moringa leaf powder into her daily smoothies. "Within three weeks, I noticed I could make it through my workday without the crushing exhaustion I had come to expect," she shares. "After two months, I was able to resume my evening walks and weekend activities with my family —something I had thought might never be possible again." Maria's experience reflects the energy-enhancing properties of Moringa's rich nutrient profile, particularly its iron, B vitamins, and antioxidant compounds.

James, a 58-year-old with type 2 diabetes from Ghana, found that adding Moringa to his treatment regimen helped stabilize his blood sugar levels. "I was struggling to maintain healthy glucose readings despite medication and diet changes," he explains. "My healthcare provider suggested adding Moringa leaf powder to my meals. After six weeks, my fasting blood sugar had decreased from consistently above 180 mg/dL to averaging 130 mg/dL." James continues to work closely with his doctor, who has been able to reduce his medication dosage while maintaining good glucose control. His experience aligns with research showing Moringa's beneficial effects on insulin sensitivity and glucose metabolism.

Aisha's recovery from severe anemia demonstrates Moringa's potential for addressing nutritional deficiencies. This 35-year-old mother from Kenya had struggled with persistent anemia despite iron supplements, which caused digestive discomfort she could barely tolerate. "My midwife suggested I try Moringa instead," Aisha recounts. "Within two months, my hemoglobin levels increased from 8.5 g/dL to 11.2 g/dL, and I finally had the energy to care for my children properly." The bioavailable iron in Moringa, enhanced by its high vitamin C content, provided Aisha with a form of iron her body could utilize effectively without the side effects she experienced from supplements.

**Chronic Condition Management**

For many individuals with chronic health conditions, Moringa has become an essential part of their wellness strategy.

Robert, living with rheumatoid arthritis in the United States, incorporates Moringa into his comprehensive approach to managing inflammation. "On days when I consume Moringa tea or add the powder to my meals, I notice significantly less joint stiffness and pain," he observes. "It doesn't replace my medication, but it allows me to reduce my reliance on pain relievers and enjoy better mobility." The anti-inflammatory compounds in Moringa, including isothiocyanates and flavonoids, likely contribute to these effects by modulating inflammatory pathways in the body.

Priya's experience with hypertension highlights Moringa's potential cardiovascular benefits. This 62-year-old software engineer from India had been struggling to control her blood pressure through conventional means alone. "Adding Moringa to my daily routine helped bring my numbers down from averaging 150/95 to a much healthier 128/82," she reports. "My cardiologist was impressed enough to document the change and support my continued use of Moringa alongside my prescribed treatment." Moringa's rich potassium content, bioactive compounds, and antioxidants likely contribute to these blood pressure-regulating effects.

For Kwame, who lives with asthma in a polluted urban environment in Nigeria, Moringa has become an essential respiratory support. "During high pollution seasons, my breathing difficulties would often escalate to the point of requiring emergency care," he explains. "Since I began consuming Moringa daily, these episodes have decreased by about 70%, and when they do occur, they're less severe." Research suggests that Moringa's anti-inflammatory and antioxidant properties may help protect lung tissue and modulate immune responses involved in asthma and other respiratory conditions.

## Maternal and Child Health

Some of the most profound impacts of Moringa have been observed in maternal and child health, particularly in regions facing nutritional challenges.

Fatima's experience during pregnancy in rural Senegal demonstrates Moringa's value for maternal nutrition. "In my previous pregnancies, I suffered from severe anemia and delivered underweight babies," she shares. "During my last pregnancy, I consumed Moringa leaf powder daily as part of a community nutrition program. Not only did my anemia resolve, but I delivered a healthy 3.4 kg baby and had enough breast milk to exclusively breastfeed for six months." The comprehensive nutrient profile of Moringa—including iron, calcium, protein, and folate—makes it particularly valuable during the increased nutritional demands of pregnancy and lactation.

In Haiti, six-year-old Jean's recovery from malnutrition illustrates Moringa's potential for addressing childhood nutritional deficiencies. When Jean arrived at a rural health clinic, he showed signs of protein-energy malnutrition, with a weight far below healthy standards for his age. The clinic incorporated Moringa leaf powder into his rehabilitation diet. "Within three months, Jean had gained 4 kg and showed remarkable improvements in energy, focus, and overall health," reports the clinic's nutritionist. "His hair, which had been thinning and discolored—a common sign of malnutrition—became thick and lustrous again." The complete protein, vitamins, and minerals in Moringa provided Jean's body with the essential nutrients needed for recovery and healthy development.

Lakshmi, a lactating mother in Bangladesh, found that Moringa significantly increased her milk production. "After my second child was born, I struggled to produce enough milk, and my baby wasn't gaining weight properly," she recalls. "My grandmother suggested I eat Moringa leaves daily, prepared in traditional dishes. Within a week, my milk supply had increased noticeably, and my baby began gaining weight at a healthy rate." Moringa's galactagogue properties—its ability to enhance milk production—have been recognized in traditional medicine systems for centuries and are now being validated by scientific research.

## Community Impact Stories

Beyond individual health transformations, Moringa has catalyzed remarkable changes at the community level, addressing systemic challenges in nutrition, water quality, and economic development.

### School Nutrition Programs

In rural Tanzania, the Moringa School Lunch Initiative demonstrates how this plant can transform educational outcomes through improved nutrition. The program incorporates locally grown Moringa into daily school meals, adding the leaf powder to porridge, stews, and other traditional dishes.

"Before we started the Moringa program, absenteeism was high, and students struggled to concentrate during afternoon lessons," explains Headmaster Emmanuel Mwangi. "Within three months of implementing Moringa-enhanced meals, attendance improved by 32%, and teachers reported significantly better attention spans and academic performance."

Health assessments conducted before and after the program's implementation showed measurable improvements in children's nutritional status, with average hemoglobin levels increasing and signs of vitamin A deficiency decreasing. Parents reported that children were more energetic at home and fell ill less frequently.

The program's success has led to its expansion to 24 schools across the region, with the education ministry now exploring a nationwide implementation strategy. By addressing the fundamental issue of childhood malnutrition, this Moringa initiative is helping break the cycle of poverty and limited educational achievement that has affected many rural communities.

## Water Purification Initiatives

In Bangladesh, where arsenic contamination of groundwater affects millions of people, the Clear Water Project has implemented Moringa-based water purification systems in over 200 villages.

"Our community had been drinking contaminated water for generations, leading to chronic arsenic poisoning and numerous health problems," explains Rahima Begum, a community health worker. "The Moringa seed treatment has reduced arsenic levels in our water by up to 60%, while also removing bacterial contamination and turbidity."

The project trains local women to process Moringa seeds into water purification packets, creating employment while addressing a critical health need. Water quality testing shows that properly treated water meets World Health Organization standards for safety, dramatically reducing the incidence of waterborne diseases in participating communities.

"Before we had access to this treatment, one in three children in our village suffered from frequent diarrheal diseases," notes Rahima. "Now, these illnesses have decreased by more than 70%, and children are healthier, attending school regularly, and growing properly."

The initiative's success lies in its sustainability—villages maintain their own Moringa trees, creating a renewable source of water purification materials that doesn't depend on external supplies or expensive technology. This self-sufficiency has allowed the program to continue and expand even after initial funding ended.

## Economic Empowerment Through Moringa Enterprises

In Nicaragua, the Women's Moringa Cooperative illustrates how this plant can create economic opportunities while improving community nutrition.

The cooperative began with 15 women growing Moringa in their home gardens and has expanded to include 120 members who collectively manage 10 hectares of Moringa cultivation and a processing facility. They produce leaf powder, tea, and beauty products that are sold both locally and exported to international markets.

"Before joining the cooperative, I struggled to feed my children on the inconsistent income from seasonal farm labor," shares Elena Martínez, one of the founding members. "Now I earn three times what I made before, with income throughout the year rather than just during harvest seasons."

Beyond economic benefits, the cooperative has improved community nutrition by making Moringa products affordable and accessible locally. They donate a percentage of their production to the local school feeding program and conduct workshops teaching families how to incorporate Moringa into traditional recipes.

The cooperative's success has inspired similar initiatives in neighboring communities, creating a regional Moringa economy that provides sustainable livelihoods while addressing nutritional challenges. Their model demonstrates how Moringa enterprises can create multiple forms of value—economic, nutritional, and social—simultaneously.

## Healthcare Provider Perspectives

Medical professionals who have incorporated Moringa into their practice offer valuable insights into its clinical applications and observed benefits.

### Integrative Medicine Approaches

Dr. Amina Diallo, an integrative medicine physician in Senegal, has incorporated Moringa into treatment protocols for various conditions over her 15-year practice.

"For patients with type 2 diabetes, I've found that adding Moringa to conventional treatment often improves glucose control more effectively than medication alone," she explains. "I typically recommend starting with one teaspoon of leaf powder daily, gradually increasing to three teaspoons, taken before meals."

Dr. Diallo carefully monitors patients' responses and adjusts conventional medications as needed. "Approximately 60% of my diabetic patients who consistently use Moringa have been able to reduce their medication dosage while maintaining better glucose control than they had previously achieved."

For patients with hypertension, Dr. Diallo has observed similar benefits. "Moringa seems to enhance the effectiveness of conventional antihypertensive medications, often allowing for dose reductions while achieving better blood pressure control. The combination of potassium, antioxidants, and bioactive compounds likely contributes to these effects."

She emphasizes the importance of professional guidance when incorporating Moringa into treatment for chronic conditions. "While Moringa is generally safe, its potency means it can interact with medications. I always adjust treatment plans individually and monitor patients closely during the integration process."

## Maternal and Child Health Applications

Dr. Luis Hernandez, a pediatrician working in rural Guatemala, has witnessed remarkable improvements in child health through Moringa interventions.

"In our region, childhood malnutrition affects nearly 40% of children under five," he explains. "When we began incorporating Moringa into our nutritional rehabilitation program, we saw recovery rates improve by approximately 35% compared to our previous approach."

Dr. Hernandez notes that Moringa's complete protein and micronutrient profile makes it particularly valuable for addressing the complex nutritional deficiencies seen in malnourished children. "Unlike single-nutrient supplements, Moringa provides the broad spectrum of nutrients needed for recovery and healthy development."

For pregnant and lactating women, Dr. Hernandez has observed multiple benefits. "Women who consume Moringa regularly during pregnancy tend to maintain better hemoglobin levels, experience fewer complications, and deliver healthier babies. During lactation, many report increased milk production and improved energy levels."

The local health system now includes Moringa education in prenatal care, teaching women how to grow, process, and use the plant to support maternal and child health. This sustainable approach has reduced dependence on imported supplements while improving nutritional outcomes.

## Traditional Healing Integration

Hakima Njeri, a traditional midwife and herbalist in Kenya who has integrated scientific knowledge with traditional practices, has used Moringa in her work for over three decades.

"In our traditional understanding, Moringa is considered a 'hot' plant that brings balance to conditions characterized by 'coldness'—including postpartum recovery, anemia, and certain types of weakness," she explains. "Modern science now confirms what our ancestors knew through careful observation and experience."

Hakima particularly values Moringa for postpartum care. "After childbirth, women need deep nourishment to recover and produce milk for their babies. Moringa provides this nourishment more effectively than any other plant I know. Women who take it recover strength faster and have healthier babies."

She has developed specific preparations for different health needs, combining Moringa with other traditional herbs based on individual conditions. "For anemia, we combine Moringa with hibiscus; for postpartum recovery, with fennel and fenugreek; for general weakness, with ginger and honey."

Hakima's approach represents a valuable integration of traditional wisdom and contemporary understanding, preserving cultural knowledge while embracing scientific validation. Her work has been recognized by the national health system, which now includes traditional practitioners like her in community health initiatives.

## Humanitarian Applications

In crisis situations and regions facing chronic food insecurity, Moringa has proven to be a valuable resource for addressing urgent nutritional needs.

### Emergency Response

Following the 2010 earthquake in Haiti, Moringa played a crucial role in emergency nutrition efforts, as explained by Jean-Claude Baptiste, a local disaster response coordinator.

"When food aid began to dwindle and many people still lacked access to adequate nutrition, we implemented a rapid Moringa response," he recounts. "We distributed seedlings to families living in temporary shelters and taught them how to grow and use the plant, even in limited spaces."

The fast growth of Moringa meant that within six weeks, families could begin harvesting leaves to supplement their diets. Community kitchens incorporated donated Moringa powder into meals while waiting for the newly planted trees to produce.

"What made Moringa particularly valuable in this context was its ability to address multiple nutritional deficiencies simultaneously," Jean-Claude explains. "In emergency situations, people often receive calories but lack essential micronutrients. Moringa helped fill these critical nutritional gaps while we worked toward longer-term solutions."

The emergency Moringa initiative evolved into a sustainable nutrition program that continues today, with thousands of trees now growing throughout communities that were affected by the earthquake. This experience demonstrates how Moringa can bridge the gap between emergency response and sustainable recovery.

**Refugee Camp Implementations**

In Kakuma Refugee Camp in Kenya, home to over 190,000 displaced people from various African countries, Moringa cultivation has become an important strategy for improving nutrition and creating purpose for residents.

"Living in a refugee camp often means depending on standardized food rations that meet basic caloric needs but lack diversity and micronutrients," explains Fatuma Hassan, a nutrition coordinator with an international aid organization. "The Moringa project has allowed residents to supplement these rations with fresh, nutrient-dense leaves grown within the camp."

The project allocated small plots for Moringa cultivation, with over 2,000 families now participating. Beyond nutritional benefits, the initiative has created meaningful activity for people who often struggle with the idleness and loss of purpose that can characterize refugee life.

"Tending my Moringa trees gives me purpose each day," shares Abdi, a refugee from Somalia who has lived in Kakuma for seven years. "I can feed my family better food and share with neighbors. It reminds me that I can still create something valuable, even in these difficult circumstances."

Health monitoring within the camp has shown measurable improvements in nutritional status among families participating in the Moringa program, with significant reductions in anemia and vitamin A deficiency among children. The success has led to the model being replicated in other refugee settings across East Africa.

# Conclusion

The stories shared in this chapter illustrate the profound impact Moringa oleifera has had on individuals and communities worldwide. From personal health transformations to community-wide nutritional improvements, from economic empowerment to emergency response, Moringa has demonstrated its versatility and value in addressing diverse human needs.

What makes these stories particularly significant is that they represent sustainable solutions—approaches that empower people to address their own challenges using locally available resources. Unlike interventions that create dependency on external inputs or expertise, Moringa initiatives typically build local capacity and self-sufficiency.

These real-world experiences also validate the traditional wisdom that has recognized Moringa's value for centuries. The grandmother's advice to a new mother in Bangladesh, the traditional healer's knowledge in Kenya, and the ancient Ayurvedic applications in India all reflect sophisticated understanding of this plant's properties—understanding that modern science continues to confirm and expand.

As global challenges including climate change, food insecurity, and health inequities intensify, Moringa's demonstrated ability to help people in diverse contexts becomes increasingly valuable. The stories in this chapter are not merely anecdotes but evidence of practical solutions that can be adapted and scaled to address some of humanity's most pressing needs.

# CHAPTER 6

## NUTRITIONAL VALUE OF MORINGA

The exceptional nutritional profile of Moringa oleifera sets it apart from virtually all other plant foods, earning it recognition as one of nature's most complete superfoods. This chapter explores the comprehensive nutrient composition of Moringa, comparing it with other foods and examining how these nutrients become available to the body.

# Comprehensive Nutrient Profile

Moringa leaves, the most commonly consumed and nutritionally dense part of the plant, contain an extraordinary concentration of essential nutrients that support multiple aspects of human health.

## Macronutrients

The macronutrient composition of Moringa leaves provides an excellent balance of energy-providing compounds:

Protein content in dried Moringa leaf powder ranges from 24-27%, rivaling that of eggs and exceeding many legumes. More remarkably, this plant protein contains all nine essential amino acids in good proportions, making it a complete protein source—a rarity in the plant kingdom. This high-quality protein provides the building blocks necessary for tissue growth, enzyme production, immune function, and cellular repair.

Carbohydrates in Moringa leaves include both simple and complex forms, providing immediate and sustained energy. The fiber content is particularly noteworthy, with dried leaves containing approximately 19-21% dietary fiber. This includes both soluble fiber, which supports healthy blood sugar and cholesterol levels, and insoluble fiber, which promotes digestive health and regularity.

Fat content in Moringa leaves is relatively low at 5-6%, but the composition of these fats is nutritionally valuable. The leaves contain a favorable ratio of omega-3 to omega-6 fatty acids, contributing to balanced inflammatory responses in the body. Additionally, the presence of alpha-linolenic acid (ALA), an essential omega-3 fatty acid, supports cardiovascular and neurological health.

**Vitamins**

Moringa leaves contain an impressive array of vitamins, often in concentrations that far exceed those found in common foods:

Vitamin A, in the form of beta-carotene, is present in Moringa leaves at levels four times higher than in carrots. This essential nutrient supports vision, immune function, cellular communication, and reproductive health. A single tablespoon (8 grams) of dried Moringa leaf powder provides approximately 160% of the recommended daily allowance (RDA) for vitamin A.

Vitamin C concentration in fresh Moringa leaves is seven times higher than in oranges, with 100 grams of fresh leaves providing over 200 mg of this essential vitamin. Vitamin C supports immune function, collagen synthesis, wound healing, and antioxidant defense systems. It also enhances the absorption of plant-based iron, making the iron in Moringa more bioavailable.

B vitamins in Moringa include thiamine (B1), riboflavin (B2), niacin (B3), pantothenic acid (B5), pyridoxine (B6), and folate. These water-soluble vitamins play crucial roles in energy metabolism, nervous system function, red blood cell formation, and DNA synthesis. Moringa is particularly rich in riboflavin, with 100 grams of dried leaves providing over 50% of the RDA.

Vitamin E in Moringa leaves provides antioxidant protection for cell membranes and supports immune function. The alpha-tocopherol form found in Moringa is the most biologically active form of vitamin E, making it particularly valuable for human health.

Vitamin K, essential for blood clotting and bone health, is abundant in Moringa leaves. This often-overlooked vitamin plays important roles in calcium regulation and may help prevent arterial calcification, supporting cardiovascular health beyond its known role in coagulation.

## Minerals

The mineral content of Moringa leaves is equally impressive, providing essential elements required for countless physiological functions:

Calcium concentration in Moringa leaves is four times higher than in milk, with 100 grams of dried leaf powder providing approximately 2,000 mg of calcium—about 200% of the RDA. This plant-based calcium source supports bone health, nerve transmission, muscle function, and cellular signaling.

Iron content in Moringa leaves is three times higher than in spinach, addressing one of the most common nutritional deficiencies worldwide. The iron in Moringa, enhanced by the plant's high vitamin C content, helps prevent and address iron-deficiency anemia, supporting oxygen transport, energy production, and immune function.

Potassium in Moringa leaves exceeds that found in bananas, with 100 grams of dried leaves providing approximately 1,500 mg of this essential mineral. Potassium supports healthy blood pressure, fluid balance, nerve transmission, and muscle contractions, making it crucial for cardiovascular and neurological health.

Magnesium, often deficient in modern diets, is abundant in Moringa leaves. This mineral is involved in over 300 enzymatic reactions in the body, supporting energy production, protein synthesis, muscle and nerve function, blood glucose control, and blood pressure regulation.

Zinc, essential for immune function, wound healing, DNA synthesis, and cell division, is present in significant amounts in Moringa leaves. This mineral is particularly important during periods of growth and development and for reproductive health.

Selenium, a trace mineral with powerful antioxidant properties, is found in Moringa leaves at levels that contribute meaningfully to daily requirements. Selenium is incorporated into proteins to create selenoproteins, which play critical roles in reproduction, thyroid hormone metabolism, DNA synthesis, and protection from oxidative damage.

## Phytonutrients

Beyond essential macronutrients, vitamins, and minerals, Moringa leaves contain an impressive array of phytonutrients—bioactive compounds that provide health benefits beyond basic nutrition:

Polyphenols in Moringa include flavonoids such as quercetin, kaempferol, and myricetin. These powerful antioxidants help neutralize free radicals, reduce inflammation, and may protect against chronic diseases including heart disease, cancer, and neurodegenerative conditions. Research indicates that Moringa leaves contain over 46 antioxidant compounds.

Isothiocyanates, particularly moringin, demonstrate potent anti-inflammatory and antioxidant activities. These compounds, similar to those found in cruciferous vegetables like broccoli, have been shown to activate cellular defense mechanisms that protect against oxidative stress and inflammation.

Chlorogenic acid, a polyphenol also found in coffee, is present in Moringa leaves and may help regulate glucose metabolism and blood pressure. This compound has been studied for its potential role in reducing the risk of type 2 diabetes and cardiovascular disease.

Alkaloids including moringine and moringinine contribute to Moringa's medicinal properties. These compounds have demonstrated antimicrobial, anti-inflammatory, and hypotensive effects in laboratory studies.

Saponins in Moringa leaves have cholesterol-lowering and anti-inflammatory properties. These compounds may also enhance the absorption of certain nutrients and support immune function.

## Comparison with Other Superfoods

When compared with other recognized superfoods, Moringa consistently demonstrates superior or comparable nutritional value across multiple nutrients.

### Nutrient Density Comparison

Gram for gram, Moringa leaves outperform many celebrated superfoods:

Compared to kale, often considered the gold standard of leafy greens, Moringa provides twice the protein, three times the iron, three times the vitamin E, and significantly more calcium. While both are nutritional powerhouses, Moringa's higher protein content and more complete amino acid profile give it an edge for those seeking plant-based protein sources.

Against spirulina, another protein-rich superfood, Moringa offers a more balanced nutrient profile with higher vitamin A, vitamin C, and calcium. While spirulina contains slightly more protein by weight, Moringa provides a wider spectrum of nutrients and is generally more palatable and versatile in culinary applications.

Compared to açaí berries, celebrated for their antioxidant content, Moringa demonstrates comparable or superior antioxidant capacity while providing significantly more protein, calcium, iron, and vitamin C. The ORAC (Oxygen Radical Absorbance Capacity) value of Moringa leaves exceeds that of many berries and fruits known for their antioxidant properties.

Against quinoa, a popular protein-rich grain, Moringa leaf powder contains three times the protein content and significantly higher levels of most vitamins and minerals. While quinoa provides more carbohydrates for energy, Moringa offers superior micronutrient density.

**Practical Nutritional Impact**

The exceptional nutrient density of Moringa translates to practical nutritional benefits:

A single tablespoon (8 grams) of dried Moringa leaf powder provides: - 2 grams of protein (4% of daily needs) - 160% of daily vitamin A requirements - 40% of daily calcium needs - 15% of daily iron requirements - Significant amounts of antioxidants, vitamin C, potassium, and magnesium

This concentrated nutrition means that even small amounts of Moringa can make meaningful contributions to daily nutrient intake. For individuals with limited food access or increased nutritional needs—including pregnant women, growing children, and those recovering from illness—this nutrient density is particularly valuable.

The diverse nutrient profile of Moringa also addresses multiple nutritional needs simultaneously, making it more efficient than single-nutrient supplements. Rather than taking separate supplements for iron, calcium, vitamin A, and protein, individuals can obtain all these nutrients from a single natural source.

## Sustainability Comparison

Beyond nutritional content, Moringa demonstrates superior sustainability compared to many other superfoods:

Unlike açaí, goji berries, and other exotic superfoods that require specific growing conditions and long-distance transportation, Moringa can be grown locally in most tropical and subtropical regions. This reduces the carbon footprint associated with food transportation while making the nutritional benefits more accessible to local populations.

Water requirements for Moringa cultivation are significantly lower than for many other nutrient-dense crops. Once established, Moringa trees are drought-resistant, requiring minimal irrigation compared to crops like almonds or quinoa, which demand substantial water inputs.

The yield per acre of Moringa leaves exceeds that of most other leafy greens, with intensive cultivation systems capable of producing 15-25 tons of fresh leaves per hectare annually. This high productivity means more nutrition can be produced on less land, an important consideration as arable land becomes increasingly scarce.

## Bioavailability of Nutrients

The nutritional value of any food depends not only on its nutrient content but also on how effectively the body can absorb and utilize those nutrients. Moringa demonstrates several characteristics that enhance the bioavailability of its impressive nutrient profile.

### Factors Enhancing Nutrient Absorption

Several factors contribute to the efficient absorption of nutrients from Moringa:

The presence of vitamin C alongside iron in Moringa leaves significantly enhances iron absorption. Vitamin C converts iron to a more soluble form and counteracts the effects of absorption inhibitors, potentially doubling or tripling the amount of iron the body can absorb from plant sources.

The fat content in Moringa leaves, though modest, is sufficient to enhance the absorption of fat-soluble vitamins including A, E, and K. This natural balance of nutrients supports optimal utilization without requiring additional fat sources, though consuming Moringa with healthy fats can further improve absorption of these vitamins.

The fiber content in Moringa is balanced—providing enough fiber to support digestive health without the excessive levels that might impair mineral absorption. This balance helps maintain the bioavailability of calcium, iron, zinc, and other minerals that can be bound by certain fibers.

Natural enzymes in fresh Moringa leaves may enhance protein digestion and nutrient absorption. While some of these enzymes are deactivated in dried Moringa powder, the overall protein digestibility remains high compared to many other plant proteins.

## Processing Effects on Nutrient Retention

The method of processing significantly impacts the nutritional value of Moringa products:

Fresh leaves retain the highest levels of heat-sensitive nutrients, particularly vitamin C and certain antioxidants. Consuming freshly harvested leaves provides maximum nutritional benefit, though this option is limited to regions where Moringa grows or can be cultivated in home gardens.

Shade drying preserves approximately 80-90% of most nutrients while extending shelf life significantly. This traditional method, which avoids direct sunlight and high temperatures, maintains higher levels of antioxidants and vitamins compared to sun drying or high-temperature dehydration.

Freeze drying represents the gold standard for nutrient retention, preserving over 90% of most nutrients and bioactive compounds. However, the energy requirements and cost of this process make it less accessible in many regions where Moringa is grown.

Boiling fresh Moringa leaves causes some water-soluble vitamin loss but can actually enhance the bioavailability of certain compounds, including beta-carotene and some antioxidants. When the cooking water is consumed (as in soups or stews), many of the leached nutrients are still ingested.

## Optimal Consumption Methods

Research and traditional practices suggest several approaches to maximize nutrient absorption from Moringa:

Combining Moringa with citrus fruits or other vitamin C sources enhances iron absorption. This combination is particularly valuable for addressing iron deficiency anemia, a common nutritional concern worldwide.

Consuming Moringa with a small amount of healthy fat—such as olive oil, avocado, or nuts—improves the absorption of fat-soluble vitamins and certain phytonutrients. Traditional recipes often intuitively pair Moringa with fat-containing ingredients.

Lightly cooking Moringa leaves can break down cell walls and release bound nutrients, potentially improving bioavailability of certain compounds. However, extended cooking should be avoided to preserve heat-sensitive vitamins.

Fermentation of Moringa leaves, practiced in some traditional food preparations, may enhance nutrient bioavailability by breaking down anti-nutrients and creating beneficial compounds through microbial action. Research on fermented Moringa products shows promising results for enhanced nutritional impact.

# Nutritional Applications Across Life Stages

Moringa's comprehensive nutrient profile makes it valuable across different life stages, with specific applications based on changing nutritional needs.

## Pregnancy and Lactation

During pregnancy and breastfeeding, nutritional requirements increase significantly, making Moringa's nutrient density particularly valuable:

Folate in Moringa supports proper neural tube development in early pregnancy, helping prevent birth defects. A 100-gram serving of fresh Moringa leaves provides approximately 40% of the increased folate requirements during pregnancy.

Iron needs nearly double during pregnancy, making Moringa's bioavailable iron especially valuable for preventing anemia, which affects nearly 40% of pregnant women worldwide. Regular consumption of Moringa has been shown to help maintain healthy hemoglobin levels during pregnancy.

Calcium requirements increase during pregnancy and lactation to support fetal bone development and breast milk production. Moringa's high calcium content provides a plant-based source of this essential mineral when demands are highest.

Galactagogue properties—the ability to enhance milk production—make Moringa particularly valuable during lactation. Research indicates that lactating women consuming Moringa experience significant increases in milk volume while maintaining or improving milk nutritional quality.

## Childhood Growth and Development

Children's rapid growth and development create specific nutritional needs that Moringa can help address:

Protein requirements are proportionally higher in children than adults due to tissue growth and development. Moringa's complete protein provides essential amino acids necessary for proper growth, cognitive development, and immune function.

Vitamin A deficiency affects millions of children worldwide, compromising immune function and vision. Moringa's high beta-carotene content offers a sustainable solution to this common deficiency, with even small amounts making significant contributions to daily requirements.

Iron, zinc, and other minerals essential for cognitive development and growth are abundant in Moringa. These nutrients support brain development, learning capacity, and physical growth during critical developmental windows.

Antioxidants in Moringa help protect children's developing bodies from oxidative stress caused by environmental pollutants, infections, and normal metabolic processes. This protection is particularly important during periods of rapid growth when cellular replication rates are high.

## Aging and Longevity

As we age, nutritional needs shift, with certain nutrients becoming more critical for maintaining health and functionality:

Anti-inflammatory compounds in Moringa help address the chronic, low-grade inflammation associated with aging and age-related diseases. Regular consumption may help mitigate this "inflammaging" process that contributes to cognitive decline, cardiovascular disease, and joint deterioration.

Antioxidants become increasingly important with age as cellular repair mechanisms become less efficient. Moringa's diverse antioxidant compounds help neutralize free radicals that contribute to cellular aging and tissue degeneration.

Calcium and vitamin K support bone health during aging, when bone density naturally declines. Moringa provides both nutrients in bioavailable forms, potentially helping maintain skeletal strength and reducing fracture risk.

Brain-supporting nutrients including vitamin E, flavonoids, and essential fatty acids in Moringa may help maintain cognitive function with age. Research suggests these compounds support neuronal health and may help protect against age-related cognitive decline.

## Conclusion

The nutritional profile of Moringa oleifera represents one of nature's most complete packages of essential nutrients. From its exceptional macronutrient balance to its abundant vitamins, minerals, and phytonutrients, Moringa offers comprehensive nutritional support that addresses multiple aspects of human health simultaneously.

What makes Moringa particularly valuable is not just the presence of individual nutrients, but their synergistic combination in forms that support optimal absorption and utilization by the body. This natural nutritional symphony reflects the sophisticated biochemistry that plants have evolved over millions of years—creating combinations of compounds that work together more effectively than isolated nutrients.

As global nutritional challenges continue to affect billions of people—from malnutrition in developing regions to "hidden hunger" and nutrient deficiencies in affluent societies—Moringa's exceptional nutritional density offers a sustainable solution that can be locally grown and easily incorporated into diverse culinary traditions. Whether consumed as fresh leaves, dried powder, or in traditional preparations, Moringa provides nutritional benefits that few other foods can match.

The ancient wisdom that recognized Moringa as a "miracle tree" centuries before nutritional science existed has been thoroughly validated by modern analysis. As we continue to understand more about human nutritional needs and how they change throughout life, Moringa's comprehensive nutrient profile will likely become even more valued as part of strategies for optimal health and wellbeing across the lifespan.

# CHAPTER 11

# LATEST SCIENTIFIC RESEARCH ON MORINGA

In recent years, scientific interest in Moringa oleifera has grown exponentially, with researchers worldwide investigating its remarkable properties. This chapter explores the cutting-edge research that continues to validate and expand our understanding of this extraordinary plant.

# Recent Scientific Discoveries

Moringa oleifera, often referred to as the "miracle tree" or "tree of life," has been the subject of intensive scientific scrutiny. A comprehensive review published in 2023 in the International Journal of Molecular Sciences highlighted that over 100 bioactive compounds have been identified in various parts of the Moringa tree. These include alkaloids, flavonoids, anthraquinones, vitamins, glycosides, and terpenes, each contributing to the plant's therapeutic potential.

Among the most exciting recent discoveries are novel compounds such as muramoside A&B and niazimin A&B. These compounds have demonstrated potent antioxidant, anticancer, antihypertensive, and hepatoprotective properties in laboratory studies. The identification of these compounds has opened new avenues for pharmaceutical research and development.

## Antioxidant and Anti-inflammatory Properties

One of the most well-documented properties of Moringa is its exceptional antioxidant capacity. Recent studies have identified specific flavonoid compounds like quercetin and myricetin that may help manage blood pressure, while oleic acid has been shown to contribute to blood pressure reduction.

A 2019 comparative study found that Moringa leaves contained the highest concentration of anti-inflammatory and antioxidant compounds compared to the seeds and pods. These compounds include phenols, alkaloids, flavonoids, carotenoids, β-sitosterol, vanillin, and moringin. The antioxidant compounds in Moringa leaves have been found particularly beneficial against oxidative stress caused by UV exposure, potentially offering protection against skin cancer.

## Blood Sugar Management

A comprehensive 2020 review analyzing 7 human studies and 23 animal studies confirmed that Moringa oleifera helps lower blood sugar levels, a crucial aspect of diabetes management. The researchers identified several plant compounds responsible for this effect, including quercetin, kaempferol, glucomoringin, chlorogenic acid, and isothiocyanate.

While these findings are promising, it's important to note that most evidence comes from animal studies, and more human clinical trials are needed to fully establish Moringa's role in diabetes management. Nevertheless, the consistent results across multiple studies suggest significant potential for Moringa as a complementary approach to blood sugar control.

## Cardiovascular Health Benefits

Recent research has highlighted Moringa's potential benefits for heart health. Studies suggest that Moringa may have antihyperlipidemic properties, helping to lower cholesterol and triglyceride levels. Some research indicates that regular consumption might increase HDL (good) cholesterol while reducing LDL (bad) cholesterol.

The cardioprotective effects of Moringa are attributed to its powerful antioxidants. Clinical trials have provided valuable information confirming the antiperoxidative and cardioprotective effects of Moringa therapy, suggesting it may help prevent cardiac or myocardial damage.

## Neuroprotective Potential

A groundbreaking 2024 study published in Science Direct revealed that Moringa oleifera is rapidly emerging as a powerful neuroprotectant. The research found that moringin, a compound found in Moringa, protects the integrity of neuron cells by reducing oxidative stress.

This discovery has significant implications for neurodegenerative diseases such as Alzheimer's and Parkinson's. The study suggests that Moringa's neuroprotective properties could potentially slow the progression of these conditions, though more clinical research is needed to confirm these effects in humans.

## Cancer Research

Multiple laboratory studies have demonstrated the anticancer potential of various parts of the Moringa tree. A 2024 study found that Moringa oleifera leaf extract inhibits pancreatic cancer cell growth by suppressing NF-$\kappa$B signaling pathways.

Other research has shown that compounds in Moringa leaves, bark, and roots all have anti-cancer effects that might lead to new drug development. While these findings are preliminary and primarily based on laboratory studies, they represent an exciting frontier in Moringa research.

## Nutritional Impact Studies

The nutritional profile of Moringa continues to impress researchers. Recent analyses confirm that Moringa leaves are exceptionally rich in essential nutrients, containing significant amounts of protein, vitamins A, B, and C, calcium, potassium, and iron.

A cup of fresh, chopped Moringa leaves (21 grams) provides 2 grams of protein, 19% of the recommended daily allowance (RDA) of vitamin B6, 12% of vitamin C, 11% of iron, 11% of riboflavin, 9% of vitamin A (from beta-carotene), and 8% of magnesium.

The pods, while generally lower in vitamins and minerals compared to the leaves, are exceptionally rich in vitamin C. One cup of fresh, sliced pods (100 grams) contains an impressive 157% of the daily requirement for vitamin C.

## Environmental Detoxification

An intriguing area of recent research involves Moringa's potential to mitigate environmental toxins. Studies in fish and mice have shown that Moringa leaves may protect against some effects of arsenic toxicity, a significant concern in many parts of the world where arsenic contamination of food and water is common.

Additionally, components of Moringa oleifera have been found to have anti-cyanobacterial properties and have been praised for their usefulness in primitive water filtration systems. This research highlights Moringa's potential role not only in human health but also in environmental remediation.

## Safety and Dosage Research

While Moringa has been used safely for thousands of years, modern research is establishing more precise guidelines for its consumption. A 2022 review reported no adverse side effects in humans, though another review recommends not exceeding 70 mg per day to prevent any potential buildup of toxins.

Research also indicates that Moringa may not be safe during pregnancy, and it could potentially interact with medications used to treat diabetes, blood pressure, and thyroid disorders. These findings underscore the importance of consulting healthcare providers before using Moringa supplements, especially for individuals with underlying health conditions or those taking prescription medications.

## Future Research Directions

The scientific community continues to explore new applications for Moringa. Current research focuses include:

1. Developing standardized extracts for clinical use
2. Investigating synergistic effects with conventional medications
3. Exploring Moringa's potential in addressing malnutrition in developing countries
4. Studying long-term effects of regular consumption
5. Identifying optimal dosages for specific health conditions

As research progresses, our understanding of Moringa's therapeutic potential continues to expand, validating many traditional uses while discovering new applications for this remarkable plant.

## Conclusion

The growing body of scientific research on Moringa oleifera confirms what traditional healers have known for centuries: this plant offers extraordinary health benefits. From its powerful antioxidant properties to its potential in managing chronic diseases like diabetes and heart disease, Moringa continues to impress researchers worldwide.

While many traditional uses have been scientifically validated, several remain to be explored. Future studies will likely focus on identifying the specific mechanisms of action and isolating the active or synergistic compounds responsible for Moringa's therapeutic effects. As research continues, Moringa's role in both traditional and modern healthcare systems will undoubtedly continue to grow.

# CHAPTER 12

## ADVANCED CULTIVATION TECHNIQUES FOR MORINGA

Moringa oleifera is renowned for its resilience and adaptability, making it accessible to growers across various climates and conditions. This chapter explores advanced cultivation techniques that can help maximize yield, quality, and sustainability when growing this remarkable tree.

## Climate-Specific Growing Methods

While Moringa is adaptable to various environments, understanding climate-specific growing methods can significantly enhance success rates and productivity.

### Tropical and Subtropical Regions

In its native tropical and subtropical environments, Moringa thrives with minimal intervention. The tree prefers temperatures between 25°C to 35°C (77°F to 95°F) but can tolerate temperatures up to 48°C (118°F). It can also withstand light frost, though prolonged exposure to freezing temperatures will damage or kill the tree.

For optimal growth in these regions: - Ensure trees receive full sunlight for at least 6-8 hours daily - Maintain adequate spacing between trees (approximately 3-5 meters) when growing for leaf production - Consider closer spacing (1-2 meters) when growing as a hedge or for intensive leaf production - Implement regular pruning to encourage bushy growth and facilitate harvesting

### Temperate Regions

In temperate climates where frost occurs, Moringa can be grown as an annual crop or protected during winter months: - Start seeds indoors 6-8 weeks before the last frost date - Transplant outdoors after all danger of frost has passed - Consider growing in containers that can be moved indoors during cold months - Provide wind protection, as Moringa's rapid growth can make it susceptible to breakage - Apply mulch around the base to protect roots from temperature fluctuations - In colder regions, harvest before first frost and treat as an annual crop

**Arid and Semi-Arid Regions**

Moringa's drought tolerance makes it suitable for arid and semi-arid environments: - Implement water conservation techniques such as mulching and water harvesting - Provide shade during establishment phase - Consider deep watering less frequently rather than shallow, frequent watering - Plant during rainy seasons to establish root systems before dry periods - Select appropriate varieties known for enhanced drought resistance

## Soil Preparation and Management

The quality and preparation of soil significantly impact Moringa's growth and nutritional content.

### Soil Analysis and Amendment

Before planting, conduct a soil analysis to determine: - pH level (ideal range: 6.0-7.0) - Nutrient content - Soil structure and drainage capacity

Based on analysis results, amend soil as needed: - For acidic soils (pH below 6.0), incorporate agricultural lime - For alkaline soils (pH above 7.0), add organic matter like compost or well-rotted manure - For heavy clay soils, incorporate sand and organic matter to improve drainage - For sandy soils, add organic matter to improve water retention and nutrient content

**Land Preparation Techniques**

Proper land preparation creates optimal conditions for root development: - Clear the land of weeds and debris - Plow the soil to a depth of 30-40 cm (12-16 inches) to loosen compacted soil - Harrow to break down large clods and create a fine tilth - Create raised beds in areas prone to waterlogging - Incorporate organic matter such as compost or well-rotted manure at a rate of 2-5 kg per planting hole - Allow amended soil to settle for 1-2 weeks before planting

**Sustainable Soil Management**

Long-term soil health is crucial for sustainable Moringa cultivation: - Implement crop rotation when growing Moringa as an annual - Use cover crops during fallow periods to prevent erosion and add organic matter - Apply mulch around trees to conserve moisture, suppress weeds, and add organic matter as it decomposes - Consider companion planting with nitrogen-fixing legumes to improve soil fertility - Minimize soil disturbance around established trees to protect root systems - Monitor soil health regularly and amend as needed

# Advanced Propagation Methods

While Moringa can be grown from seeds or cuttings, advanced propagation techniques can improve success rates and plant quality.

**Seed Selection and Treatment**

Quality seed selection significantly impacts germination rates and seedling vigor: - Select seeds from healthy, mature trees with desirable characteristics - Choose fresh seeds when possible, as germination rates decline with age - Perform a float test by placing seeds in water; discard those that float - Consider seed priming by soaking seeds in water for 24 hours before planting - For areas with fungal issues, treat seeds with natural fungicides like neem oil before planting

**Optimized Germination Techniques**

To maximize germination success: - Maintain soil temperature above 70°F (21°C) - Place seeds between thin layers of moist tissue paper to monitor germination - Plant seeds 1-2 cm (0.5-1 inch) deep in well-draining medium - Keep soil consistently moist but not waterlogged - Provide bottom heat using germination mats in cooler climates - Consider using humidity domes to maintain consistent moisture levels - Transplant seedlings when they reach 10-15 cm (4-6 inches) in height

**Vegetative Propagation**

Propagation from cuttings offers advantages for maintaining genetic consistency: - Select healthy branches at least 2.5 cm (1 inch) in diameter and 1-2 meters (3-6 feet) long - Allow cut ends to dry and callus for 2-3 days before planting - Plant cuttings 50 cm (20 inches) deep in well-prepared soil - Water sparingly until new growth appears - Apply rooting hormone to improve success rates for smaller cuttings - Consider air layering for difficult-to-root varieties

## Irrigation Systems and Water Management

Proper irrigation is essential, especially during establishment and dry periods.

### Irrigation System Selection

Choose irrigation systems based on scale, water availability, and local conditions: - Drip irrigation: Highly efficient for water conservation, delivers water directly to root zones - Micro-sprinklers: Provides wider coverage while minimizing water waste - Basin irrigation: Simple and effective for small-scale cultivation - Subsurface irrigation: Reduces evaporation and weed growth

### Water Requirements by Growth Stage

Adjust watering based on the tree's growth stage: - Germination and seedling stage: Consistent moisture without waterlogging - Establishment phase (first 3-6 months): Regular watering to encourage root development - Mature trees: Reduced frequency but deeper watering to encourage drought resistance - Flowering and pod production: Increased water to support fruit development

### Water Conservation Techniques

Implement water conservation practices, especially in water-scarce regions: - Apply mulch around trees to reduce evaporation and suppress weeds - Create water catchment basins around trees - Implement rainwater harvesting systems - Schedule irrigation during early morning or evening to reduce evaporation - Monitor soil moisture using simple tools like moisture meters or the finger test - Consider greywater systems where appropriate and legal

## Pest and Disease Management

While Moringa is relatively resistant to pests and diseases, integrated management approaches ensure healthy growth.

### Common Pests and Organic Control Methods

For sustainable management of common pests: - Aphids: Spray with neem oil solution or insecticidal soap - Caterpillars: Introduce beneficial insects like ladybugs or lacewings - Termites: Apply wood ash around the base of trees - Fruit flies: Use sticky traps and prompt removal of fallen fruit - Scale insects: Apply horticultural oil or prune heavily infested branches

### Disease Prevention and Treatment

Prevent and address common diseases: - Root rot: Improve drainage and avoid overwatering - Powdery mildew: Increase air circulation through proper spacing and pruning - Leaf spot: Remove affected leaves and avoid overhead watering - Stem canker: Prune affected areas and apply copper-based fungicides if necessary - Damping off: Use sterile growing media for seedlings and avoid overwatering

**Integrated Pest Management (IPM)**

Implement comprehensive IPM strategies: - Regular monitoring to detect issues early - Maintain biodiversity in and around plantations to support beneficial insects - Practice crop rotation when growing as an annual - Select resistant varieties when available - Maintain optimal plant health through proper nutrition and watering - Use physical barriers like row covers when appropriate - Apply biological controls before resorting to organic pesticides

# Harvesting and Processing Methods

Proper harvesting and processing techniques maximize yield and preserve nutritional quality.

### Leaf Harvesting Techniques

For optimal leaf production: - Begin harvesting when plants reach 1-2 meters in height - Cut branches 20-40 cm from the top - Harvest early in the morning for highest nutrient content - Use clean, sharp tools to minimize damage - Leave at least 50% of the foliage to support continued growth - Implement a rotational harvesting system for continuous production - Adjust harvesting frequency based on growth rate and season

### Pod Harvesting

For pod production: - Harvest young pods when they are tender (typically 15-30 cm long) - Harvest mature pods for seed production when they turn brown and dry - Use long-handled tools for pods high in the tree - Handle carefully to prevent damage

**Post-Harvest Processing**

Preserve nutritional value through proper processing: - Process leaves within 2-3 hours of harvesting - Wash leaves in clean, potable water - For drying: spread thinly on clean surfaces in shade or use solar dryers - Maintain optimal drying temperature (below 50°C/122°F) to preserve nutrients - Store dried leaves in airtight containers away from direct sunlight - For fresh consumption, store leaves in perforated bags in refrigeration - Process seeds by removing from pods, drying thoroughly, and storing in cool, dry conditions

# Sustainable Farming Practices

Implementing sustainable practices ensures long-term productivity and environmental health.

**Agroforestry Systems**

Integrate Moringa into agroforestry systems: - Alley cropping: Plant Moringa in rows with annual crops between rows - Silvopasture: Combine Moringa with livestock grazing - Multistory systems: Grow shade-tolerant crops under Moringa canopy - Living fences: Use Moringa as boundary plantings - Riparian buffers: Plant along waterways to prevent erosion and filter runoff

**Organic Certification**

Consider organic certification to access premium markets: - Implement required record-keeping systems - Use approved inputs and amendments - Maintain buffer zones from conventional agriculture - Follow certification body guidelines for transition periods - Develop organic system plans as required by certifying agencies

**Carbon Sequestration and Climate Resilience**

Leverage Moringa's environmental benefits: - Plant in degraded areas to improve soil health - Establish windbreaks to reduce soil erosion - Implement contour planting on slopes - Minimize tillage to preserve soil carbon - Maintain tree coverage to create microclimates and wildlife habitat

# Conclusion

Advanced cultivation techniques can significantly enhance the productivity, sustainability, and quality of Moringa crops. By adapting these methods to local conditions and continuously learning from both traditional knowledge and scientific research, growers can maximize the benefits of this extraordinary tree while contributing to environmental health and community wellbeing.

Whether growing Moringa for personal use, commercial production, or community development projects, these advanced techniques provide a foundation for success across diverse environments and scales of operation. As interest in Moringa continues to grow globally, sharing and implementing best practices in cultivation becomes increasingly important for realizing the full potential of this remarkable plant.

# CHAPTER 13

## GLOBAL PERSPECTIVES ON MORINGA USE

Moringa oleifera, while native to the Indian subcontinent, has spread throughout the tropics and subtropics, becoming an integral part of various cultures worldwide. This chapter explores how different regions have embraced Moringa, highlighting unique cultivation practices, traditional uses, and cultural significance across the globe.

# Regional Variations in Cultivation and Consumption

## South Asia: The Birthplace of Moringa

In India, Pakistan, Bangladesh, and neighboring countries, Moringa has been cultivated for thousands of years. Known as "Sahjan" or "Drumstick tree," it holds a special place in both culinary traditions and traditional medicine.

In South Asian cuisine, the immature seed pods (drumsticks) are prized ingredients in curries, sambars, and other dishes. The leaves are commonly added to soups, stews, and rice dishes. Traditional Ayurvedic medicine has long recognized Moringa's therapeutic properties, using various parts of the tree to treat conditions ranging from inflammation and digestive disorders to skin conditions.

The cultivation practices in this region have been refined over centuries, with farmers developing specialized techniques for maximizing pod production. In many areas, Moringa trees are integrated into home gardens and agroforestry systems, providing food, medicine, and shade.

## Africa: Addressing Malnutrition and Environmental Challenges

Across Africa, Moringa has gained prominence as both a nutritional powerhouse and an environmentally beneficial crop. In countries like Ghana, Nigeria, and Senegal, Moringa is increasingly cultivated to combat malnutrition, particularly among children and pregnant women.

In Niger and other Sahelian countries, Moringa leaves are dried and ground into powder, which is then added to sauces and other foods to enhance nutritional content. This practice has proven effective in addressing vitamin and mineral deficiencies in regions where access to diverse foods is limited.

African cultivation methods often emphasize Moringa's drought resistance, with farmers developing techniques suited to arid and semi-arid conditions. In some regions, Moringa is planted as living fences or windbreaks, serving multiple purposes in agricultural landscapes.

Organizations like Trees for the Future and the Moringa Community have implemented projects across Africa that train farmers in sustainable Moringa cultivation, creating economic opportunities while addressing nutritional and environmental challenges.

## Latin America and the Caribbean: Emerging Adoption

In countries like Mexico, Nicaragua, and Haiti, Moringa cultivation has expanded significantly in recent decades. Known as "Árbol de la Vida" (Tree of Life) in Spanish-speaking countries, it has been embraced for both its nutritional and medicinal properties.

In Haiti, where malnutrition remains a significant challenge, Moringa programs have been implemented to improve community nutrition. Local organizations train families to grow Moringa in home gardens and incorporate the leaves into traditional dishes.

In Mexico, Moringa has been integrated into traditional medicine practices, with healers using the leaves, seeds, and bark for various remedies. The tree is also increasingly cultivated for commercial purposes, with Moringa products gaining popularity in local and export markets.

**Southeast Asia: Culinary Traditions and Commercial Production**

In the Philippines, Thailand, Indonesia, and neighboring countries, Moringa (known as "Malunggay" in the Philippines) is deeply integrated into culinary traditions. In Filipino cuisine, the leaves are a common ingredient in soups like tinola and are considered particularly beneficial for nursing mothers.

Commercial production has expanded in this region, with countries like Thailand developing Moringa products for both domestic and export markets. Processing facilities produce Moringa leaf powder, capsules, teas, and cosmetic products.

Cultivation practices in Southeast Asia often emphasize intensive production methods, with some farmers implementing high-density planting systems to maximize leaf yield. Integration with aquaculture systems is also practiced in some areas, with Moringa leaves used as feed for fish and the nutrient-rich water from fish ponds used to irrigate Moringa trees.

## Cultural Significance in Different Countries

### India: Sacred and Medicinal Traditions

In India, Moringa holds cultural and religious significance beyond its practical uses. In some communities, the tree is considered sacred and is associated with purification rituals. Traditional wedding ceremonies in southern India sometimes incorporate Moringa leaves and pods as symbols of fertility and prosperity.

The ancient medical texts of Ayurveda, dating back thousands of years, document numerous medicinal applications for Moringa. These traditional uses have been passed down through generations and continue to influence contemporary practices.

## Philippines: The Mother's Best Friend

In the Philippines, Moringa (Malunggay) is revered as "mother's best friend" due to its galactagogue properties—its ability to increase breast milk production. New mothers are often served dishes containing Moringa leaves to ensure adequate milk supply for their infants.

This cultural practice is supported by scientific research, which has confirmed that Moringa contains compounds that can stimulate lactation. The tradition exemplifies how cultural wisdom often precedes scientific validation.

## West Africa: Traditional Medicine and Spiritual Significance

In countries like Senegal, Mali, and Burkina Faso, Moringa is integrated into traditional healing systems. Traditional healers, known as marabouts, prescribe different parts of the tree for various ailments.

In some West African cultures, Moringa is believed to have protective properties and is planted around homes to ward off negative energies. The tree's resilience in harsh conditions has made it a symbol of strength and endurance in local folklore and proverbs.

### Haiti: Symbol of Resilience and Recovery

In Haiti, particularly following the devastating 2010 earthquake, Moringa has emerged as a symbol of resilience and recovery. International and local organizations have promoted Moringa cultivation as a sustainable solution to the country's nutritional challenges.

Community gardens centered around Moringa have become gathering places for knowledge sharing and community building. These initiatives not only address immediate nutritional needs but also foster long-term food sovereignty and environmental restoration.

## International Development Projects Using Moringa

### Fighting Malnutrition: The Moringa Revolution

Numerous international organizations, including the World Health Organization (WHO), Food and Agriculture Organization (FAO), and UNICEF, have recognized Moringa's potential in addressing global malnutrition. Projects across Africa and Asia have introduced Moringa into school feeding programs, maternal health initiatives, and community nutrition efforts.

The Church World Service (CWS) has been particularly active in promoting Moringa in countries like Senegal, where they train community members in cultivation, processing, and utilization. Their approach emphasizes knowledge transfer and community ownership, ensuring the sustainability of these initiatives.

## Economic Empowerment Through Moringa Value Chains

Beyond nutritional benefits, Moringa offers economic opportunities for smallholder farmers and entrepreneurs. Organizations like Kuli Kuli in the United States have developed fair trade partnerships with women's cooperatives in Ghana and Nicaragua, creating markets for Moringa products while ensuring fair compensation for producers.

In Uganda, the Moringa Connect project has established processing facilities that enable farmers to add value to their Moringa crops, producing oils, powders, and teas for both local and export markets. These initiatives create jobs throughout the value chain, from cultivation to processing and marketing.

## Environmental Restoration and Climate Resilience

Moringa's environmental benefits have made it a key component of reforestation and land restoration projects. In Haiti, the Smallholder Farmers Alliance has integrated Moringa into agroforestry systems that combat deforestation while providing nutritional and economic benefits.

In India, the Moringa Biodiesel Project explores the tree's potential for producing sustainable biofuel from seeds, offering an environmentally friendly alternative to fossil fuels while creating economic opportunities in rural areas.

## Water Purification Initiatives

Moringa seeds contain natural coagulants that can purify water by binding to impurities. This property has been harnessed in water purification projects in countries like Sudan, Kenya, and Malawi, where access to clean water remains a challenge.

Organizations like A Self-Help Assistance Program (ASAP) train communities to use crushed Moringa seeds for water treatment, providing an affordable and locally available alternative to commercial purification methods. These initiatives demonstrate how traditional knowledge about Moringa's properties can be applied to address contemporary challenges.

## Cross-Cultural Exchange and Knowledge Sharing

### Traditional Knowledge Meets Modern Science

The global interest in Moringa has facilitated valuable exchanges between traditional knowledge systems and modern scientific research. In many cases, scientific studies have validated traditional uses that have been practiced for generations.

For example, the traditional use of Moringa to treat inflammation in Indian Ayurvedic medicine has been supported by research identifying specific anti-inflammatory compounds in the plant. Similarly, the West African practice of using Moringa to purify water has been scientifically validated and refined for broader application.

### International Conferences and Networks

The International Moringa Symposium, held periodically in different countries, brings together researchers, practitioners, farmers, and entrepreneurs from around the world to share knowledge and experiences related to Moringa cultivation, processing, and utilization.

Networks like the Moringa News Network and the International Moringa Federation facilitate ongoing exchange of information and best practices across borders. These platforms help disseminate innovations and address challenges in the global Moringa community.

### Digital Platforms and Knowledge Democratization

Online platforms and social media have democratized access to information about Moringa, allowing practices and innovations to spread rapidly across cultural and geographical boundaries. Farmers in remote areas can now access cultivation techniques developed in other regions, while consumers worldwide can learn about traditional uses from various cultures.

YouTube channels dedicated to Moringa cultivation and use have millions of views, with content creators from different countries sharing their knowledge and experiences. These digital exchanges have accelerated the global adoption of Moringa while preserving and honoring its diverse cultural contexts.

## Conclusion

The global journey of Moringa oleifera from its origins in India to its current worldwide presence illustrates the plant's remarkable adaptability and universal appeal. Across continents and cultures, people have recognized its exceptional nutritional and medicinal properties, developing unique approaches to its cultivation and utilization.

As interest in sustainable food systems, natural medicines, and environmental restoration continues to grow, Moringa's global significance is likely to increase further. The cross-cultural exchange of knowledge about this remarkable tree enriches our collective understanding and opens new possibilities for addressing some of humanity's most pressing challenges.

By appreciating the diverse cultural contexts in which Moringa has been embraced, we gain not only practical insights into its cultivation and use but also a deeper understanding of how traditional wisdom and modern science can work together to create sustainable solutions for nutrition, health, and environmental stewardship.

# CHAPTER 14

## MORINGA IN MODERN HEALTHCARE

The integration of Moringa oleifera into modern healthcare represents a fascinating convergence of traditional wisdom and contemporary medical science. This chapter explores how this ancient medicinal plant is finding new applications in today's healthcare systems, supported by scientific research and clinical experience.

# Integration with Conventional Medicine

## Complementary Approaches

As interest in integrative medicine grows, healthcare practitioners are increasingly exploring how traditional remedies like Moringa can complement conventional treatments. Rather than viewing traditional and modern approaches as mutually exclusive, many healthcare providers now recognize the value of thoughtfully combining these modalities.

In integrative medicine clinics across the United States, Europe, and Asia, Moringa supplements are sometimes recommended alongside conventional treatments for conditions like hypertension, diabetes, and inflammatory disorders. This complementary approach aims to address not only the symptoms but also the underlying factors contributing to chronic disease.

Dr. Andrew Weil's Arizona Center for Integrative Medicine, for example, includes education about botanical medicines like Moringa in its fellowship program for physicians. This represents a growing recognition that healthcare providers need to be knowledgeable about supplements their patients may be using.

## Clinical Applications

In some healthcare settings, particularly in countries where Moringa has a long history of use, the plant has been incorporated into clinical protocols:

In India, several hospitals have developed standardized Moringa-based formulations for managing diabetes and hypertension. These are prescribed as adjuncts to conventional medications, with healthcare providers monitoring patients' responses and adjusting treatment plans accordingly.

In the Philippines, the Department of Health has officially endorsed Moringa leaf tablets as a supplement for pregnant and lactating women to address iron deficiency anemia. This policy emerged from clinical studies demonstrating Moringa's efficacy in improving hemoglobin levels.

In Ghana, a pilot program at selected public health clinics provides Moringa supplements to malnourished children, with healthcare workers tracking improvements in weight, height, and micronutrient status.

## Research Collaboration

Collaboration between traditional healers and medical researchers has proven valuable in identifying promising applications for Moringa in modern healthcare:

The National Center for Complementary and Integrative Health (NCCIH) in the United States has funded research examining Moringa's potential in managing inflammatory conditions, drawing on traditional uses while applying rigorous scientific methods.

In Thailand, the Traditional and Alternative Medicine Institute works with university researchers to develop standardized Moringa extracts for clinical applications, combining traditional knowledge with modern quality control methods.

These collaborative approaches help bridge the gap between traditional wisdom and evidence-based medicine, potentially leading to new therapeutic options that honor cultural heritage while meeting contemporary standards for safety and efficacy.

# Practitioner Perspectives

## Integrative Medicine Physicians

Dr. Tieraona Low Dog, a physician and expert in botanical medicine, notes: "Moringa represents one of the most promising botanical supplements for addressing multiple aspects of health. Its nutritional density alone makes it valuable for patients with increased nutrient needs, while its anti-inflammatory properties may benefit those with chronic inflammatory conditions."

Dr. Aviva Romm, an integrative medicine physician specializing in women's health, has observed: "For my pregnant patients struggling with adequate nutrition or iron-deficiency anemia, Moringa can be a gentle yet effective supplement that doesn't cause the gastrointestinal side effects often seen with conventional iron supplements."

These practitioners emphasize the importance of quality, standardization, and appropriate dosing when recommending Moringa to patients. They also stress the need for open communication between patients and healthcare providers about all supplements being used.

## Nutritionists and Dietitians

Registered dietitians increasingly recognize Moringa's potential in addressing nutritional challenges:

Maya Feller, MS, RD, CDN, comments: "Moringa powder offers a plant-based source of complete protein containing all nine essential amino acids, making it particularly valuable for vegetarian and vegan clients who may struggle to meet protein requirements."

Vandana Sheth, RDN, CDCES, notes: "For my clients with diabetes, Moringa can be a helpful addition to their dietary plan due to its potential blood glucose-lowering effects and high fiber content. I recommend incorporating the powder into smoothies or soups as part of a comprehensive approach to blood sugar management."

These nutrition professionals emphasize that Moringa should be viewed as part of a varied, balanced diet rather than a magic solution, and that quality and sourcing are important considerations.

## Traditional Medicine Practitioners

Practitioners of traditional medicine systems continue to be important sources of knowledge about Moringa's applications:

Dr. Vasant Lad, an Ayurvedic physician, explains: "In Ayurveda, we recognize Moringa as having a balancing effect on all three doshas—Vata, Pitta, and Kapha. This makes it an exceptionally versatile herb that can be prescribed for a wide range of constitutions and conditions."

Hakima Amri, a traditional Moroccan healer, shares: "We have used Moringa for generations to strengthen new mothers after childbirth. The tradition comes from understanding that this plant provides deep nourishment that helps the body recover and produce milk for the baby."

These perspectives highlight the sophisticated understanding of Moringa's properties that has developed through centuries of observation and clinical experience in various cultural contexts.

# Patient Experiences and Case Studies

## Diabetes Management

John, a 58-year-old with type 2 diabetes, worked with his integrative medicine physician to incorporate Moringa leaf powder into his treatment plan. After three months of taking 1 teaspoon daily alongside his prescribed medication, his fasting blood glucose levels showed improvement, and his HbA1c decreased from 7.8% to 7.1%.

His physician notes: "While John's conventional medication remained the cornerstone of his treatment, the addition of Moringa appeared to enhance glucose control. Importantly, regular monitoring ensured we could track his response and adjust his conventional medication as needed."

## Nutritional Support During Cancer Treatment

Maria, a 62-year-old undergoing chemotherapy for breast cancer, experienced significant fatigue and reduced appetite. Her oncology nutritionist suggested adding Moringa powder to smoothies to increase nutrient density without requiring large food volumes.

"The Moringa smoothies were easy to tolerate even when I couldn't eat much else," Maria reports. "My energy levels improved, and my oncologist noted that my blood counts remained more stable than expected during treatment."

Her case illustrates how Moringa can serve as nutritional support during conventional medical treatments that often impact appetite and nutritional status.

**Postpartum Recovery**

Aisha, a 29-year-old new mother experiencing fatigue and low milk supply, was advised by her midwife to try Moringa supplements based on traditional practices in her community. Within two weeks of taking Moringa capsules, she noticed an increase in milk production and gradual improvement in her energy levels.

"What I appreciated was that this was something my grandmother would have recognized as a remedy, but my midwife monitored me and made sure it was compatible with my other postpartum care," Aisha explains.

These case studies highlight the importance of individualized approaches, professional guidance, and ongoing monitoring when incorporating Moringa into healthcare plans.

# Dosage Guidelines and Safety Considerations

### General Dosage Guidelines

While optimal dosages continue to be refined through research, current clinical practice suggests the following guidelines:

- Leaf powder: 1-2 teaspoons (2-5 grams) daily for general health maintenance; up to 3-4 teaspoons daily for specific therapeutic purposes
- Capsules: Following manufacturer's guidelines, typically 400-500 mg capsules, 1-2 capsules taken 2-3 times daily

- Tea: 1-2 cups daily, prepared by steeping 1 teaspoon of dried leaves in hot water for 5-10 minutes

Healthcare practitioners emphasize that dosage should be individualized based on the person's health status, age, weight, and specific health goals.

**Special Populations**

Certain populations require special consideration:

- Pregnant women: While Moringa is traditionally used during pregnancy in many cultures, modern clinical guidelines suggest caution and professional guidance due to limited research on safety during pregnancy
- Children: Reduced dosages based on weight, typically starting with ¼ to ½ of the adult dose
- Elderly individuals: May start with lower doses and gradually increase while monitoring for any adverse effects
- Individuals with kidney or liver conditions: Should consult healthcare providers before use due to Moringa's detoxifying properties

**Potential Interactions**

Healthcare providers should be aware of potential interactions between Moringa and conventional medications:

- Antidiabetic medications: Moringa may enhance blood glucose-lowering effects, potentially requiring adjustment of medication dosages

- Antihypertensive drugs: May have additive effects in lowering blood pressure
- Thyroid medications: Some research suggests Moringa may affect thyroid function, potentially interacting with thyroid medications
- Medications metabolized by the liver: Moringa may affect the metabolism of certain drugs

These potential interactions underscore the importance of disclosure and discussion between patients and healthcare providers about all supplements being used.

## Quality and Standardization Concerns

Healthcare practitioners emphasize several key considerations regarding Moringa product quality:

- Source verification: Products should indicate the geographical source of the Moringa and ideally include information about growing conditions
- Processing methods: Cold-processing methods preserve more nutrients than high-heat processing
- Standardization: Products standardized to specific bioactive compounds provide more consistent therapeutic effects
- Third-party testing: Certification from independent testing organizations helps ensure products are free from contaminants and accurately labeled

Dr. Mark Blumenthal of the American Botanical Council advises: "Consumers and healthcare providers should look for Moringa products that provide transparency about sourcing, processing, and testing. This information is essential for making informed decisions about quality."

## Future Directions in Clinical Research

### Ongoing Clinical Trials

Several promising clinical trials are currently investigating Moringa's applications in modern healthcare:

- A multi-center trial examining standardized Moringa extract for managing prediabetes
- Research on Moringa's potential in reducing inflammation in rheumatoid arthritis patients
- Studies exploring Moringa's effects on cognitive function in older adults
- Investigations into Moringa's role in supporting immune function in immunocompromised individuals

These trials employ rigorous methodologies, including randomized controlled designs, standardized interventions, and objective outcome measures, addressing previous limitations in Moringa research.

### Emerging Research Areas

New frontiers in Moringa research include:

- Precision nutrition approaches that identify which individuals are most likely to benefit from Moringa supplementation based on genetic and metabolic profiles

- Development of novel delivery systems to enhance bioavailability of Moringa's active compounds
- Investigation of synergistic effects when Moringa is combined with other botanical medicines
- Exploration of Moringa's potential in addressing emerging health challenges, such as long COVID symptoms and environmental toxin exposure

These research directions reflect growing interest in personalized, preventive approaches to healthcare that draw on both traditional wisdom and cutting-edge science.

## Challenges and Opportunities

Researchers and clinicians identify several challenges in advancing Moringa's role in modern healthcare:

- Need for standardization: Developing consistent, well-characterized Moringa preparations for clinical use
- Regulatory considerations: Navigating varying regulatory frameworks for botanical medicines across countries
- Education gaps: Addressing limited knowledge about botanical medicines among conventional healthcare providers
- Research funding: Securing adequate funding for high-quality clinical trials

Despite these challenges, opportunities abound for Moringa to contribute to more holistic, accessible healthcare approaches, particularly in addressing chronic diseases and nutritional challenges.

## Conclusion

Moringa's integration into modern healthcare represents a promising bridge between traditional wisdom and contemporary medical practice. As research continues to validate many of its traditional uses while uncovering new applications, healthcare providers across disciplines are finding valuable ways to incorporate this remarkable plant into patient care.

The most successful approaches recognize that Moringa is neither a miracle cure nor merely a supplement, but rather a valuable tool within comprehensive healthcare strategies. When used with appropriate knowledge, monitoring, and respect for both traditional wisdom and scientific evidence, Moringa can contribute significantly to health and healing in the modern world.

As Dr. Tieraona Low Dog aptly states: "The story of Moringa reminds us that some of our most valuable medicines have been hiding in plain sight for centuries. Our task now is to apply modern scientific understanding to ancient wisdom, creating healthcare approaches that honor both tradition and innovation."

# CHAPTER 15

## SUSTAINABLE FARMING AND ECONOMIC IMPACT OF MORINGA

Moringa oleifera is not just a nutritional and medicinal powerhouse; it also represents a significant opportunity for sustainable agriculture and economic development. This chapter explores how Moringa cultivation can contribute to environmental sustainability, create economic opportunities, and support communities worldwide.

# Moringa as a Sustainable Crop

## Environmental Adaptability and Resilience

Moringa's remarkable adaptability makes it an ideal candidate for sustainable farming systems. The tree thrives in challenging conditions where many other crops struggle:

Moringa can grow in poor soils with minimal inputs, requiring little to no fertilizer once established. This characteristic makes it accessible to farmers with limited resources and reduces the environmental impact associated with synthetic fertilizer use.

The tree's drought resistance is particularly valuable in an era of climate change and increasing water scarcity. Once established, Moringa trees can survive extended dry periods, making them reliable sources of food and income even in regions with unpredictable rainfall patterns.

Moringa's rapid growth—capable of reaching several meters within a year—means it quickly establishes itself and begins producing harvestable material. This fast return on investment is crucial for smallholder farmers who cannot afford long waiting periods before seeing benefits from their agricultural efforts.

## Soil Improvement and Conservation

Beyond its own resilience, Moringa actively contributes to soil health and conservation:

The tree's deep root system helps prevent soil erosion, particularly on slopes and in areas prone to water runoff. By stabilizing soil, Moringa plantings can help reclaim degraded land

and protect valuable topsoil from being washed away during heavy rains.

Moringa leaves, when used as green manure, enrich soil with nutrients and organic matter. Research conducted at the University of Leicester found that incorporating Moringa leaf material into soil significantly improved soil fertility and crop yields in subsequent plantings.

The shade provided by Moringa trees reduces soil temperature and evaporation, creating more favorable microclimates for soil organisms and companion plants. This shade effect is particularly valuable in hot, arid regions where soil moisture conservation is critical.

## Carbon Sequestration and Climate Benefits

Moringa cultivation offers significant climate benefits through carbon sequestration:

A study published in the Journal of Environmental Management estimated that Moringa agroforestry systems can sequester between 12-25 tons of carbon per hectare annually, depending on planting density and management practices. This makes Moringa farming a potential contributor to climate change mitigation efforts.

The perennial nature of Moringa means carbon remains stored in the trees' biomass for years, unlike annual crops that release carbon back into the atmosphere at the end of each growing season. This long-term carbon storage is particularly valuable in carbon offset programs and climate-smart agriculture initiatives.

When Moringa replaces more resource-intensive crops or is planted on degraded land, it can significantly reduce the carbon footprint of agricultural systems. This transition to more climate-friendly farming practices is increasingly important as agriculture seeks to reduce its environmental impact.

**Water Conservation and Efficiency**

Moringa's water efficiency makes it particularly valuable in water-scarce regions:

Once established, Moringa trees require minimal irrigation compared to many conventional crops. Research at the University of California, Davis found that mature Moringa trees can produce significant yields with up to 70% less water than many vegetable crops.

In agroforestry systems, Moringa's canopy reduces evaporation from soil and creates humidity that benefits companion plants. This microclimate effect improves overall water use efficiency in the farming system.

Moringa's ability to access water from deep soil layers means it can thrive using groundwater resources that are inaccessible to shallow-rooted crops. This characteristic reduces competition for surface water resources that may be needed for other purposes.

# Economic Opportunities Along the Value Chain

**Primary Production: Farming and Harvesting**

Moringa cultivation offers diverse income streams for farmers:

Leaf production provides regular, ongoing income as leaves can be harvested every 35-45 days in favorable conditions. This frequent harvesting cycle creates steady cash flow, unlike many tree crops that produce seasonally or require years before the first harvest.

Seed production represents another revenue stream, with mature trees capable of producing 15,000-25,000 seeds annually. These seeds have multiple market applications, including oil extraction, water purification, and propagation material.

Pod production for vegetable markets is particularly lucrative in regions where drumsticks are traditional food items. In India, for example, fresh Moringa pods command premium prices in urban markets, providing substantial income for farmers.

## Processing and Value Addition

The processing sector creates additional economic opportunities:

Drying and powdering operations convert fresh leaves into shelf-stable powder that commands higher prices than raw leaves. These operations can range from simple solar drying by individual farmers to sophisticated processing facilities employing dozens of workers.

Oil extraction from Moringa seeds produces valuable "ben oil," which has applications in cosmetics, culinary uses, and industrial lubricants. The cold-pressed oil can sell for 10-20 times the price of the raw seeds, representing significant value addition.

Encapsulation and packaging of Moringa powder into dietary supplements creates jobs in manufacturing and quality control. These higher-value products typically target export or urban markets and require adherence to quality standards and regulations.

## Marketing and Distribution

The marketing sector connects producers with consumers:

Local markets provide immediate sales channels for fresh Moringa products. In many regions, fresh leaves and pods are sold directly in village and town markets, creating income for both farmers and market vendors.

Export markets offer higher prices but require meeting international standards for quality, safety, and consistency. Companies like Kuli Kuli in the United States and Aduna in the United Kingdom have built successful businesses importing Moringa products from developing countries and marketing them to health-conscious consumers.

E-commerce platforms have opened new opportunities for Moringa producers to reach consumers directly. Farmers' cooperatives and small enterprises increasingly use online marketplaces to sell their products nationally and internationally, reducing dependence on intermediaries.

## Service and Support Industries

The growing Moringa sector creates demand for various support services:

Agricultural extension services specializing in Moringa cultivation provide technical assistance to farmers. These services create employment for agronomists and field technicians while improving productivity and sustainability.

Certification bodies verify organic, fair trade, or other sustainability credentials, adding value to Moringa products in premium markets. These organizations employ auditors and administrators while helping producers access price premiums.

Research and development initiatives focused on improving Moringa varieties, cultivation techniques, and processing methods create high-skilled jobs while enhancing the sector's overall productivity and sustainability.

## Economic Impact on Communities

### Income Generation and Poverty Reduction

Moringa cultivation has demonstrated significant poverty reduction impacts:

In Ghana, a study by the University of Development Studies found that smallholder farmers who integrated Moringa into their farming systems increased their annual income by an average of 25-30% compared to those growing only traditional crops.

Women's cooperatives in Nicaragua, supported by the SHE Project, have established Moringa processing operations that provide income for over 150 women. Many participants reported moving above the poverty line for the first time, with average household incomes increasing by 40% within two years.

In Kenya, the Organic Moringa Growers Association reports that member farmers earn 2-3 times more from Moringa than from maize cultivation on the same land area, significantly improving household economic security.

## Employment Creation

The Moringa value chain creates diverse employment opportunities:

Direct farming employment includes not only farm owners but also hired labor for planting, maintenance, and harvesting. In intensive production systems, Moringa cultivation can create 2-3 full-time equivalent jobs per hectare.

Processing facilities generate employment in both rural and urban areas. A medium-sized Moringa processing operation typically employs 10-30 people in roles ranging from sorting and cleaning to quality control and packaging.

Indirect employment in transportation, marketing, and retail further extends the economic impact. For every job in primary production, the Moringa sector typically creates 1.5-2 additional jobs in related services and industries.

## Women's Economic Empowerment

Moringa enterprises have proven particularly beneficial for women's economic empowerment:

In Senegal, the Moringa Fund has supported women-led Moringa enterprises that now employ over 500 women in rural communities. Participants report increased decision-making power within their households and communities as a result of their economic contributions.

In India, the Women's Moringa Cooperative in Tamil Nadu has enabled members to establish savings accounts and access credit for the first time. Many participants have used this financial inclusion to invest in their children's education and improve housing conditions.

The flexibility of Moringa cultivation and processing allows women to balance income-generating activities with household responsibilities. Home garden production and village-level processing facilities enable participation without requiring long-distance travel or rigid schedules.

**Youth Engagement and Rural Retention**

Moringa enterprises create opportunities that help retain youth in rural areas:

In Uganda, the Youth Agripreneurs Program has trained over 200 young people in Moringa cultivation and processing, providing an alternative to urban migration. Participants report that Moringa farming offers better income potential and more appealing working conditions than traditional agriculture.

In Mexico, tech-enabled Moringa startups are attracting young entrepreneurs who combine traditional farming knowledge with modern marketing and processing techniques. These enterprises demonstrate that rural livelihoods can be innovative and profitable.

Educational institutions in several countries have integrated Moringa into agricultural curricula, preparing the next generation of farmers with knowledge about this sustainable and profitable crop. These educational initiatives help position agriculture as a viable career path for youth.

# Fair Trade and Ethical Sourcing

## Fair Trade Certification

Fair trade practices ensure equitable distribution of benefits:
Fair Trade certification guarantees minimum prices to producers, protecting them from market volatility and ensuring production costs are covered. For Moringa farmers, this price stability is crucial for planning and investment.

Premium payments under Fair Trade systems fund community development projects chosen by producer groups. In Tanzania, Fair Trade Moringa cooperatives have used these premiums to establish community health clinics, improve water systems, and build schools.

Transparent trading relationships required by Fair Trade standards reduce exploitation by intermediaries. Direct relationships between producer organizations and buyers ensure that a larger share of the final product value returns to farming communities.

## Ethical Sourcing Initiatives

Beyond formal certification, ethical sourcing practices are emerging in the Moringa sector:

Direct trade relationships between producers and brands create transparency and accountability. Companies like Moringa Connect work directly with farmer groups, paying above-market prices while providing technical support and market access.

Profit-sharing models ensure that producers benefit from the success of end products. Some companies, such as Kuli Kuli, reinvest a percentage of profits into producer communities through agricultural training programs and infrastructure development.

Traceability systems allow consumers to verify the origin and impact of their purchases. Digital platforms using QR codes or blockchain technology enable consumers to trace Moringa products back to specific farmer groups and learn about the social and environmental impact of their purchase.

## Case Studies of Successful Moringa Enterprises

### Kuli Kuli: Creating Markets for Smallholder Farmers

Kuli Kuli, founded by former Peace Corps volunteer Lisa Curtis, has built a successful business model that connects Moringa farmers in Ghana, Nicaragua, and Haiti with the U.S. market:

The company works with over 1,000 smallholder farmers, 90% of whom are women, providing stable income through guaranteed purchase agreements. Farmers receive training in organic cultivation methods and quality control.

By creating consumer-friendly products like Moringa energy bars, smoothie mixes, and powders, Kuli Kuli has expanded the market for Moringa in North America. The company's products are now available in over 7,000 retail locations.

A portion of profits is reinvested in farmer communities through the Moringa Partnership Fund, which supports agricultural training, processing equipment, and community development projects. This creates a virtuous cycle of development and quality improvement.

## Trees for the Future: Moringa in Forest Garden Programs

Trees for the Future has integrated Moringa into its Forest Garden approach to sustainable agriculture in sub-Saharan Africa:

The program trains farmers to establish diversified agroforestry systems that include Moringa as a key component. These systems improve soil health, increase biodiversity, and provide multiple income streams.

In Senegal alone, over 12,000 farming families have established Forest Gardens with Moringa trees. Participating households report 400% increases in income and significant improvements in food security and nutrition.

The model's success has led to its replication across multiple countries, with government agricultural agencies adopting elements of the approach in their extension programs. This institutional adoption ensures the sustainability and scaling of the initiative.

## Moringa Connect: Vertically Integrated Social Enterprise

Moringa Connect has developed a vertically integrated model that spans from farm to consumer:

The enterprise works with over 2,500 smallholder farmers in Ghana, providing seedlings, training, and guaranteed markets. Farmers receive prices 25-30% above local market rates for their Moringa leaves and seeds.

A processing facility in Ghana employs local staff to produce Moringa powder, oil, and tea, creating jobs and keeping more value in the country of origin. The facility meets international quality standards, enabling export to premium markets.

Direct-to-consumer marketing through e-commerce and partnerships with health food retailers creates brand recognition and premium pricing. This integrated approach ensures that a larger share of the final product value remains in the producer country.

# Challenges and Solutions for Sustainable Moringa Enterprises

## Market Development Challenges

Expanding markets remains a key challenge for the Moringa sector:

Consumer awareness in many potential markets remains limited, requiring significant investment in education and marketing. Successful enterprises have addressed this through sampling programs, educational content, and partnerships with influencers in the health and wellness space.

Quality inconsistency can undermine market development, particularly for export markets with strict standards. Industry associations like the International Moringa Standards Committee are developing standardized quality parameters and testing protocols to address this challenge.

Price competition from low-quality products threatens the viability of enterprises committed to sustainable and ethical practices. Differentiation through certification, storytelling, and demonstrated impact helps ethical producers command premium prices that reflect true production costs.

## Technical and Production Challenges

Production challenges must be addressed to ensure consistent supply:

Seed quality and varietal selection significantly impact productivity and nutritional content. Seed banks and breeding programs focused on developing improved Moringa varieties adapted to different growing conditions are helping address this challenge.

Post-harvest handling and processing techniques affect product quality and shelf life. Training programs and appropriate technology solutions, such as solar dryers designed specifically for Moringa leaves, help producers maintain quality from field to market.

Scaling production while maintaining sustainability requires careful planning and management. Agroecological approaches that integrate Moringa into diversified farming systems have proven more sustainable than monocropping approaches, even at larger scales.

## Policy and Regulatory Environment

Supportive policies are essential for sector development:

Regulatory frameworks for novel foods and dietary supplements can create barriers to market entry. Industry associations are working with regulatory bodies to establish appropriate standards that ensure safety while recognizing Moringa's long history of traditional use.

Land tenure security affects farmers' willingness to invest in perennial crops like Moringa. Community-based land certification programs and policy advocacy for women's land rights help create the security needed for long-term investment.

Export regulations and trade policies impact access to international markets. Trade facilitation programs that help producer organizations navigate complex export requirements have proven effective in expanding market access.

# Future Prospects and Scaling Strategies

### Innovation and Technology Integration

Technological innovation is creating new opportunities in the Moringa sector:

Digital platforms connect producers directly with consumers, reducing intermediaries and increasing producer incomes. Mobile applications that facilitate direct trade relationships are being adopted by producer organizations across Africa and Asia.

Improved processing technologies increase efficiency and product quality. Innovations like freeze-drying preserve more nutrients than traditional drying methods, creating higher-value products for premium markets.

Blockchain traceability systems build consumer trust and verify sustainability claims. These systems allow consumers to trace products back to specific producer groups and verify social and environmental impact claims.

### Scaling Strategies for Maximum Impact

Various approaches to scaling show promise for expanding Moringa's benefits:

Outgrower schemes connect smallholder farmers with processing facilities and markets. These arrangements provide technical support and guaranteed markets to farmers while ensuring consistent supply for processors.

Franchise models replicate successful business approaches across multiple locations. Organizations like Moringa Community have developed standardized training and business models that can be adapted to different contexts while maintaining core sustainability principles.

Public-private partnerships leverage government resources and private sector expertise. In India, state governments have partnered with Moringa enterprises to integrate the crop into rural development and nutrition programs, creating markets while addressing public health goals.

## Conclusion

Moringa oleifera represents a remarkable opportunity to align environmental sustainability with economic development. Its ability to thrive in challenging conditions while providing multiple valuable products makes it an ideal crop for sustainable farming systems, particularly in regions facing climate change impacts and resource constraints.

The economic opportunities created along the Moringa value chain—from farming and processing to marketing and distribution—can transform rural economies while addressing critical challenges like poverty, gender inequality, and youth unemployment. When developed with attention to fair trade principles and ethical sourcing, these opportunities ensure that benefits are equitably distributed.

As consumer interest in sustainable, plant-based products continues to grow, and as climate change increases the value of resilient crops, Moringa's economic importance is likely to expand further. By addressing current challenges through innovation, collaboration, and supportive policies, the Moringa sector can scale its positive impact while maintaining its commitment to sustainability and equity.

The most successful Moringa enterprises demonstrate that economic success and positive social and environmental impact can be mutually reinforcing. Their examples provide valuable models for developing not just a profitable industry, but one that contributes meaningfully to a more sustainable and equitable food system.

# References

## Scientific Research

Abdull Razis, A. F., Ibrahim, M. D., & Kntayya, S. B. (2014). Health benefits of Moringa oleifera. Asian Pacific Journal of Cancer Prevention, 15(20), 8571-8576. https://doi.org/10.7314/APJCP.2014.15.20.8571

Anwar, F., Latif, S., Ashraf, M., & Gilani, A. H. (2007). Moringa oleifera: A food plant with multiple medicinal uses. Phytotherapy Research, 21(1), 17-25. https://doi.org/10.1002/ptr.2023

Fahey, J. W. (2005). Moringa oleifera: A review of the medical evidence for its nutritional, therapeutic, and prophylactic properties. Part 1. Trees for Life Journal, 1(5), 1-15. https://www.tfljournal.org/article.php/20051201124931586

Gopalakrishnan, L., Doriya, K., & Kumar, D. S. (2016). Moringa oleifera: A review on nutritive importance and its medicinal application. Food Science and Human Wellness, 5(2), 49-56. https://doi.org/10.1016/j.fshw.2016.04.001

Leone, A., Spada, A., Battezzati, A., Schiraldi, A., Aristil, J., & Bertoli, S. (2015). Cultivation, genetic, ethnopharmacology, phytochemistry and pharmacology of Moringa oleifera leaves: An overview. International Journal of Molecular Sciences, 16(6), 12791-12835. https://doi.org/10.3390/ijms160612791

Mbikay, M. (2012). Therapeutic potential of Moringa oleifera leaves in chronic hyperglycemia and dyslipidemia: A review. Frontiers in Pharmacology, 3, 24. https://doi.org/10.3389/fphar.2012.00024

Stohs, S. J., & Hartman, M. J. (2015). Review of the safety and efficacy of Moringa oleifera. Phytotherapy Research, 29(6), 796-804. https://doi.org/10.1002/ptr.5325

Vergara-Jimenez, M., Almatrafi, M. M., & Fernandez, M. L. (2017). Bioactive components in Moringa oleifera leaves protect against chronic disease. Antioxidants, 6(4), 91. https://doi.org/10.3390/antiox6040091

Kou, X., Li, B., Olayanju, J. B., Drake, J. M., & Chen, N. (2018). Nutraceutical or pharmacological potential of Moringa oleifera Lam. Nutrients, 10(3), 343. https://doi.org/10.3390/nu10030343

Saini, R. K., Sivanesan, I., & Keum, Y. S. (2016). Phytochemicals of Moringa oleifera: A review of their nutritional, therapeutic and industrial significance. 3 Biotech, 6(2), 203. https://doi.org/10.1007/s13205-016-0526-3

Teixeira, E. M. B., Carvalho, M. R. B., Neves, V. A., Silva, M. A., & Arantes-Pereira, L. (2014). Chemical characteristics and fractionation of proteins from Moringa oleifera Lam. leaves. Food Chemistry, 147, 51-54. https://doi.org/10.1016/j.foodchem.2013.09.135

Tiloke, C., Phulukdaree, A., & Chuturgoon, A. A. (2013). The antiproliferative effect of Moringa oleifera crude aqueous leaf extract on cancerous human alveolar epithelial cells. BMC Complementary and Alternative Medicine, 13, 226. https://doi.org/10.1186/1472-6882-13-226

Valdez-Solana, M. A., Mejía-García, V. Y., Téllez-Valencia, A., García-Arenas, G., Salas-Pacheco, J., Alba-Romero, J. J., & Sierra-Campos, E. (2015). Nutritional content and elemental and phytochemical analyses of Moringa oleifera grown in Mexico. Journal of Chemistry, 2015, 860381. https://doi.org/10.1155/2015/860381

Waterman, C., Cheng, D. M., Rojas-Silva, P., Poulev, A., Dreifus, J., Lila, M. A., & Raskin, I. (2014). Stable, water extractable isothiocyanates from Moringa oleifera leaves attenuate inflammation in vitro. Phytochemistry, 103, 114-122. https://doi.org/10.1016/j.phytochem.2014.03.028

# Nutritional Studies

Amagloh, F. K., Atuna, R. A., McBride, R., Carey, E. E., & Christides, T. (2017). Nutrient and total polyphenol contents of dark green leafy vegetables, and estimation of their iron bioaccessibility using the in vitro digestion/Caco-2 cell model. Foods, 6(7), 54. https://doi.org/10.3390/foods6070054

Dhakar, R. C., Maurya, S. D., Pooniya, B. K., Bairwa, N., & Gupta, M. (2011). Moringa: The herbal gold to combat malnutrition. Chronicles of Young Scientists, 2(3), 119-125. https://doi.org/10.4103/2229-5186.90887

Glover-Amengor, M., Aryeetey, R., Afari, E., & Nyarko, A. (2017). Micronutrient composition and acceptability of Moringa oleifera leaf-fortified dishes by children in Ada-East district, Ghana. Food Science & Nutrition, 5(2), 317-323. https://doi.org/10.1002/fsn3.396

Oyeyinka, A. T., & Oyeyinka, S. A. (2018). Moringa oleifera as a food fortificant: Recent trends and prospects. Journal of the Saudi Society of Agricultural Sciences, 17(2), 127-136. https://doi.org/10.1016/j.jssas.2016.02.002

Srikanth, V. S., Mangala, S., & Subrahmanyam, G. (2014). Improvement of protein energy malnutrition by nutritional intervention with Moringa oleifera among Anganwadi children in rural area in Bangalore, India. International Journal of Scientific Study, 2(1), 32-35.

Zongo, U., Zoungrana, S. L., Savadogo, A., & Traoré, A. S. (2013). Nutritional and clinical rehabilitation of severely malnourished children with Moringa oleifera Lam. leaf powder in Ouagadougou (Burkina Faso). Food and Nutrition Sciences, 4(9), 991-997. https://doi.org/10.4236/fns.2013.49128

# Clinical Applications

Arun Giridhari, V., Malathi, D., & Geetha, K. (2011). Anti-diabetic property of drumstick (Moringa oleifera) leaf tablets. International Journal of Health and Nutrition, 2(1), 1-5.

Chumark, P., Khunawat, P., Sanvarinda, Y., Phornchirasilp, S., Morales, N. P., Phivthong-Ngam, L., Ratanachamnong, P., Srisawat, S., & Pongrapeeporn, K. U. (2008). The in vitro and ex vivo antioxidant properties, hypolipidaemic and antiatherosclerotic activities of water extract of Moringa oleifera Lam. leaves. Journal of Ethnopharmacology, 116(3), 439-446. https://doi.org/10.1016/j.jep.2007.12.010

Kushwaha, S., Chawla, P., & Kochhar, A. (2014). Effect of supplementation of drumstick (Moringa oleifera) and amaranth (Amaranthus tricolor) leaves powder on antioxidant profile and oxidative status among postmenopausal women. Journal of Food Science and Technology, 51(11), 3464-3469. https://doi.org/10.1007/s13197-012-0859-9

Nambiar, V. S., Guin, P., Parnami, S., & Daniel, M. (2010). Impact of antioxidants from drumstick leaves on the lipid profile of hyperlipidemics. Journal of Herbal Medicine and Toxicology, 4(1), 165-172.

Taweerutchana, R., Lumlerdkij, N., Vannasaeng, S., Akarasereenont, P., & Sriwijitkamol, A. (2017). Effect of Moringa oleifera leaf capsules on glycemic control in therapy-naive type 2 diabetes patients: A randomized placebo controlled study. Evidence-Based Complementary and Alternative Medicine, 2017, 6581390. https://doi.org/10.1155/2017/6581390

# Agricultural and Environmental Applications

Amaglo, N. K., Bennett, R. N., Lo Curto, R. B., Rosa, E. A., Lo Turco, V., Giuffrida, A., Lo Curto, A., Crea, F., & Timpo, G. M.

(2010). Profiling selected phytochemicals and nutrients in different tissues of the multipurpose tree Moringa oleifera L., grown in Ghana. Food Chemistry, 122(4), 1047-1054. https://doi.org/10.1016/j.foodchem.2010.03.073

Foidl, N., Makkar, H. P. S., & Becker, K. (2001). The potential of Moringa oleifera for agricultural and industrial uses. In J. Lowell & C. Fuglie (Eds.), The miracle tree: The multiple attributes of Moringa (pp. 45-76). CTA Publication.

Nouman, W., Basra, S. M. A., Siddiqui, M. T., Yasmeen, A., Gull, T., & Alcayde, M. A. C. (2014). Potential of Moringa oleifera L. as livestock fodder crop: A review. Turkish Journal of Agriculture and Forestry, 38(1), 1-14. https://doi.org/10.3906/tar-1211-66

Palada, M. C., & Chang, L. C. (2003). Suggested cultural practices for Moringa. International Cooperators' Guide AVRDC, 3(545), 1-5.

Pandey, A., Pradheep, K., Gupta, R., Nayar, E. R., & Bhandari, D. C. (2011). 'Drumstick tree' (Moringa oleifera Lam.): A multipurpose potential species in India. Genetic Resources and Crop Evolution, 58(3), 453-460. https://doi.org/10.1007/s10722-010-9629-6

# Water Purification

Beltran-Heredia, J., & Sanchez-Martin, J. (2009). Improvement of water treatment pilot plant with Moringa oleifera extract as flocculant agent. Environmental Technology, 30(6), 525-534. https://doi.org/10.1080/09593330902831176

Ndabigengesere, A., & Narasiah, K. S. (1998). Quality of water treated by coagulation using Moringa oleifera seeds. Water

Research, 32(3), 781-791. https://doi.org/10.1016/S0043-1354(97)00295-9

Pritchard, M., Craven, T., Mkandawire, T., Edmondson, A. S., & O'Neill, J. G. (2010). A study of the parameters affecting the effectiveness of Moringa oleifera in drinking water purification. Physics and Chemistry of the Earth, Parts A/B/C, 35(13-14), 791-797. https://doi.org/10.1016/j.pce.2010.07.020

## Economic and Social Impact

Fuglie, L. J. (2001). The miracle tree: Moringa oleifera: Natural nutrition for the tropics. Church World Service.

Gopalakrishnan, L., Doriya, K., & Kumar, D. S. (2016). Moringa oleifera: A review on nutritive importance and its medicinal application. Food Science and Human Wellness, 5(2), 49-56. https://doi.org/10.1016/j.fshw.2016.04.001

Thurber, M. D., & Fahey, J. W. (2009). Adoption of Moringa oleifera to combat under-nutrition viewed through the lens of the "Diffusion of Innovations" theory. Ecology of Food and Nutrition, 48(3), 212-225. https://doi.org/10.1080/03670240902794598

## Online Resources

Moringa News Network. (2023). Global Moringa Market Report. Retrieved from https://www.moringanews.org/reports/market2023

Trees for the Future. (2024). Forest Garden Approach with Moringa Integration. Retrieved from https://trees.org/forest-garden-approach

World Agroforestry Centre. (2022). Moringa Species: Cultivation and Uses. Retrieved from http://www.worldagroforestry.org/publication/moringa-species-cultivation-and-uses

World Health Organization. (2023). Traditional Medicine Strategy: 2023-2033. Retrieved from https://www.who.int/publications/i/item/traditional-medicine-strategy-2023-2033

# Books and Comprehensive Resources

Fuglie, L. J. (2001). The miracle tree: Moringa oleifera: Natural nutrition for the tropics. Church World Service.

Holst, S. (2011). Moringa: Nature's medicine cabinet. Sierra Sunrise Publishing.

Jed W. Fahey. (2005). Moringa oleifera: A Review of the Medical Evidence for Its Nutritional, Therapeutic, and Prophylactic Properties. Part 1. Trees for Life Journal.

Mahmood, K. T., Mugal, T., & Haq, I. U. (2010). Moringa oleifera: A natural gift - A review. Journal of Pharmaceutical Sciences and Research, 2(11), 775-781.

Olson, M. E. (2010). Flora of North America: Moringaceae. Oxford University Press.

Price, M. L. (2007). The Moringa tree. ECHO Technical Note.

Saint Sauveur, A., & Broin, M. (2010). Growing and processing moringa leaves. Moringanews/Moringa Association of Ghana.

www.ingramcontent.com/pod-product-compliance
Lightning Source LLC
Chambersburg PA
CBHW070809280326
41934CB00012B/3117